AF540442

Artificial Insemination in Goats

NIPA® GENX ELECTRONIC RESOURCES & SOLUTIONS P. LTD.
New Delhi-110 034

About the Editors

Dr Chetna Gangwar was born on 10.11.1982 in Distt Pilibhit of Uttar Pradesh. Dr Gangwar worked as veterinary officer in Department of Animal Husbandry, U.P. from 22.12.2007 to 31.12.2012. Then she gets selected in ARS and became scientist in ICAR on 1.1.2013. Dr Gangwar is currently working as scientist in Animal Physiology and Reproduction Division, ICAR-CIRG, Mathura. Dr Gangwar did her B.V.Sc in 2006 with 85.17% marks and M.V.Sc in Animal Reproduction with 87.28% marks in 2008 from G.B.P.U.A & T, Pantnagar, Uttarakhand. Dr Gangwar completed her Ph.D. in 2017 with 88.88% marks from DUVASU, Mathura. Dr Gangwar has published 61 research articles in the journals of national and international repute. Along with this she has developed one Mobile App on "Artificial insemination in goats", commercialized 4 technology, one on "Goat semen diluents composition and cryopreservation protocol", published 4 books, 28 book chapters, 7 manuals, 8 folders, 47 technical articles, delivered 4 radio talks and 3 T.V. talk and guided 5 students. Dr Gangwar has worked in 15 research projects as either PI or Co-PI, Dr Gangwar has organized many training programmes, like 1 winter school sponsored by ICAR, 1 workshop sponsored by SERB, 22 National training programmes on "Scientific goat farming", 8 specialized training programmes on "Artificial Insemination in Goats", 9 Sponsored training programmes on "Goat farming" and organized as well as attended various Kisan Melas, Kisan Gosthis, Field days, Awareness Camps etc. Dr Gangwar has received many prestigious awards from international and national societies, like Associate fellowship from National Academy of Dairy Sciences (NADSI) 2022, Prof. S.S. Guraya Young Scientist Award 2022 from ISSRF, Dr Vallabh Mandokot Young Woman Veterinarian Award 2020 from National Academy of Veterinary Sciences (NAVS), Scientist Award of ISSAR in 2014, 8 Best Oral Presentation Awards, Many Best Paper Awards and Excellent Reviewer Award etc. Dr Gangwar is working in the area of buck semen cryopreservation and is eminent scientist of male reproduction. Dr Gangwar is member of editorial board of "Livestock Research International Journal", E-Pashupalan an online magazine, Annual Report of CIRG, Ajamukh (Newsletter) of CIRG etc. from last 4 years as well as she is reviewer of many international journals like Reproduction in Domestic Animals, Andrologia, Theriogenology, Asian Pacific Journal of Reproduction, Veterinary Research Communications, Indian Journal of Animal Sciences, Indian Journal of Small Ruminants etc.

Dr. S.D. Kharche was born in 1962 in Madhya Pradesh state. He graduated in Veterinary Science and Animal Husbandry from Mhow Veterinary College in 1986. He received his Master's degree in Veterinary Gynaecology and Obstetrics in 1989 and Doctorate degree in 1998 from Deemed University, IVRI Izatnagar (U.P.).

Dr. Kharche started his professional career in 1989 at Indian Veterinary Redearch Institute, Izatnagar. Soon he joined as Chief Veterinary Officer cum Project Manager in 1990 at Dairy Farm of Korakundah Estate, Ooty, TNAU. After qualifying the Agriculture Research Services of ICAR, he joined as Scientist, at NAARM, Hyderabad in 1992 and soon he joined as Scientist, Animal Reproduction at IVRI Izatnagar in 1993. Later he was selected and joined as Senior Scientist, Animal Reproduction in 2001 Principal scientist from 01-01-2009 and is continuing as Incharge APR Division, ICAR-CIRG Makhdoom from 01-08-2019 till date.

Dr. Kharche in his professional career has made enormous scientific contributions in Reproductive Biotechnology. He did significant work on Oestrus Synchronization, Multiple Ovulation and Embryo Transfer in Cattle and Goat and develop new superovulation protocol. He has been instrumental in the team for production of calves and kids through Embryo Transfer, production of kid through IVM, IVF and IVC and production of several calves and kids through Artificial Insemination. As reproduction scientist he has made significant contributions In Reproductive herd health management and treatment of reproductive disorders in Cattle, Buffalo, Sheep and Goat. During his tenure infrastructure development and Re modeling of laboratory took place.

Dr. Kharche has been an active researcher and worked in 28 research projects as PI and CO-PI and has to his credit with 150 papers published in national and international journals, 85 popular articles, one technical bulletin and edited 5 books. He has guided 22 students and 01 post-doc.

Dr. Kharche nominated by ICAR as an expert for training on A.I. and goat management to Zambia. and visited Argentina to attend and present research papers in 36th Annual conference of International Embryo transfer Society.

Dr. Kharche is recipient of Junior and Senior Research Fellowship and several professional awards: Prof. Nil's lagerlof Memorial Award – 2001, G. B. Singh Memorial Award – 2003, Gaon Gyan Paritoshik Award – 2006, and several awards for Hindi shodh patra presentation in Hindi Pakhwada. Beside this he is also recipient of ISSGPR Fellow-2019, NAVS Fellow-2019 and ISSAR Fellow-2019.

R. Pourouchottamane is presently working as a Principal Scientist (LPM) at ICAR-Central Institute for Research on Goats, Makhdoom, Mathura (U.P.). He had his graduation in Veterinary Sciences and Animal Husbandry from Madras Veterinary College (TANUVAS) and did his Master's and Doctoral degree in Livestock Production Management from VCRI, Namakkal (TANUVAS) and ICAR-IVRI, Izatnagar in 1999 and 2001, respectively. He has 20 years of experience in various fields of animal production system like pig husbandry (ICAR-NRC on Pig, Guwahati), yak husbandry (ICAR-NRC on Yak, Dirang), sheep and rabbit farming (ICAR-CSWRI), goat husbandry (ICAR-CIRG, Makhdoom) as well as on farming system Research (ATARI, Barapani). He has published more than 80 research papers and popular articles in various national and international journals of repute. He has published books on different species and farming system research like Scientific Pig Production and Management: A Bio-treasure for Rural Society (IBPSS, New Delhi), Technology inventory for livestock and poultry production in North Eastern Region (ZC Unit, Zone3, Meghalaya), Handbook on Commercial Goat (ICAR-CIRG) and Goat Husbandry and Management (ICAR RC for NEH region, Meghalaya).

Dr. Ravi Ranjan born on December 11,1979, obtained BVSc & AH from WBUAFS, Kolkata, M.V.Sc. from NDRI, Karnal, Haryana and PhD from IVRI, Bareilly, UP. After joining as Scientist in Indian Council for Agriculture Research in 2007 at ICAR-CIRG, Mathura, UP, he became Senior Scientist in 2017 and continuing. He is renowned Scientist in the area of Reproductive Physiology and Biotechnology. He had published more than 65 research papers in National and International reputed Journal. He had published 03 books 10 Training Manual and more than 100 book chapters. He has completed more than 12 Research project and presently handling 08 research project as PI and Co-PI from different funding agency (DBT, DST, NABARD, ICAR, NLM, AICRP etc.). He had standardized and developed semen freezing protocol and Artificial Insemination techniques in different breeds of goats and produced more than 500 kids at this Institute and this Technology was commercialised and Transferred to Aegidan Animal Biocare Pvt. Ltd. Hooghly, W.B. India. He has guided 4 B.Sc., 2 M.Sc and presently 3 PhD students are working. He has successfully organized 30 trainings, 2 workshop/ symposia including International Conference and workshop, 02 ICAR winter course, Entrepreneurship Development Programmes, Model Training Courses, and Industry- Farmer Interface etc. He is recipients of several awards in his name, NAAS Associate Fellow Award, NADSI Associate Fellow Award, S. C. Sud Memorial Best Thesis Award, S. S. Guraya Young Scientist Award, Young Scientist Award (SURE), Best oral and poster Presentation Award, D. N. Pandey best poster Award etc. He also started training in Goat semen freezing and AI Training to different stakeholder and started commercialization of goat semen straws first time in India from ICAR Institute.

Artificial Insemination in Goats

Chetna Gangwar
Senior Scientist (Animal Reproduction)
Animal Physiology and Reproduction Division
ICAR- Central Institute for Research on Goats
Makhdoom, Mathura, Uttar Pradesh

S.D. Kharche
Principal Scientist (Animal Reproduction)
Animal Physiology and Reproduction Division
ICAR- Central Institute for Research on Goats
Makhdoom, Mathura, Uttar Pradesh

R. Pourouchottamane
Principal Scientist (Livestock Production & Management)
Animal Physiology and Reproduction Division
ICAR- Central Institute for Research on Goats
Makhdoom, Mathura, Uttar Pradesh

Ravi Ranjan
Senior Scientist (Animal Physiology)
Animal Physiology and Reproduction Division
ICAR- Central Institute for Research on Goats
Makhdoom, Mathura, Uttar Pradesh

NIPA® GENX ELECTRONIC RESOURCES & SOLUTIONS P. LTD.
New Delhi-110 034

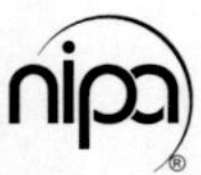

NIPA® GENX ELECTRONIC RESOURCES & SOLUTIONS P. LTD.

101,103, Vikas Surya Plaza, CU Block
L.S.C.Market, Pitam Pura, New Delhi-110 034
Ph : +91 11 27341616, 27341717, 27341718
E-mail:newindiapublishingagency@gmail.com
www: www.nipabooks.com

For customer assistance, please contact
Phone: + 91-11-27 34 17 17
Fax: + 91-11-27 34 16 16
E-Mail: feedbacks@nipabooks.com

ISBN: 978-93-95763-17-2

Composed and Designed by NIPA®.

Foreword

Small ruminants are the mainstay of arid, semiarid and rain fed agro ecosystem of the country and carry tremendous potential to contribute to rural livelihood and economy of developing nations like India owing to its short production cycle, quick returns as well as premium quality meat. Out of 148.88 million total goats in India, around 63.5 per cent are of non-descript nature, while 27.4 per cent are pure and 9.1 per cent are graded goats. There is a huge scope to improve the production potential of non-descript goats through introduction of elite males from purebreds native to the region or from adjoining region. The selection of breeding animals in relation to maximizing the reproductive efficiency depends upon males selected for breeding. Artificial Insemination permits intense selection of sires with exceptional merits and provides opportunity to exploit the value of superior sires. This book constitutes an update of recent developments in the field of assisted reproductive technology which includes selection and management of breeding buck, semen collection, processing and cryopreservation, estrous synchronization and Artificial insemination, pregnancy diagnosis and quality control in Artificial Insemination. Recently in some of these fields remarkable progress has been made. None the less, imperfections are remaining and sustained efforts will be required to optimize existing techniques and invent the new ones. The recent progress made on ART is covered in this book. I congratulate the authors for compiling this manual to be used by the trainees. I am sure that it would enrich the knowledge of the students and trainees in the field of ART not only limited to goats but also in sheep husbandry. The learners will have better understanding and pave the way for use of these techniques for enhancing the socio- economic benefits of goat enterprise in the national economy.

-sd-

Director ICAR-CIRG

Contents

1

Artificial Insemination in Goats: An Overview

Chetna Gangwar, Ravi Ranjan and Manish K. Chatli

Division of AP&R, ICAR- Central Institute for Research on Goats Makhdoom, Farah-281122, Mathura, Uttar Pradesh

Globally there is growing demand for small ruminant production especially, goats for meat and milk purposes to feed the ever-increasing human population. As per 20th Livestock Census released by Department of Animal Husbandry & Dairying, the Goat population in the country in 2019 is **148.88 million** showing an increase of **10.1%** over the previous census Out of 148.88 million Indigenous Goats (Including Non-descript), 27.4% are pure breed, 9.1% are graded breeds and the remaining 63.5% are non-descript breeds. The goat population has increased at a faster growth rate in India and varied from 0.94 to 5.10% with an average of 3.05% during 1951-2013 in spite of about 41% slaughter and about 15% natural annual mortality. India produced 21.71% of the milk, 10.47% of the meat and 13.15% of the fresh skins of the world goat production worth of Rs. 1,06,335 million per annum. The goat husbandry also generates about 4.2% rural employment over 500,000 remote villages. It contributes nearly 8.5% of the total GDP from livestock sector to Indian agriculture production system. So, to increase the productivity per goat, we need to improve the breed quality scientifically.

Traditionally, goat breeding is based on natural mating which possesses certain risks of sexually transmitted diseases and accumulation of recessive traits causing inbreeding depression. Artificial insemination (AI) offers an alternative to traditional breeding methods. AI has an important role in goat breeding, especially in intensive production systems to control reproduction and improve meat, milk and fibre production. Various factors are responsible for the success rate of AI in goats like impact of cryopreservation on semen, bacterial load, and semen quality. The place of deposition of semen also plays a major role in conception rate which improves with the depth of insemination. There are four techniques of artificial insemination viz., vaginal, intracervical, trans-cervical and laparoscopic intrauterine insemination. Vaginal insemination involves 2 High End Workshop on Advances in Artificial Insemination in Goats

deposition of semen in cranial part of vagina. This technique is not widely practiced as it requires higher sperm concentration in semen for insemination and also results in poor conception rates (5 to 20%); however, intracervical insemination is widely used in goats and is easy to perform within 2 to 3 min and conception rate depends on depth of penetration. Intravaginal and intracervical inseminations are commonly used by most of the inseminators.

Table 1: Comparison of methods of artificial insemination in goats

S.No.	Methods of A.I. in goats	No of sperm required	Time required	Conception rate
1.	Vaginal	More than the methods listed at 2, 3, & 4	Least (< 1 min)	Least (0-20%)
2.	Intracervical	Less no of sperm	Lesser (1-2 min)	Lesser (up to 57%)
3.	Trans-cervical	Lesser no of sperm	Less (> 2 min)	High (up to 71%)
4.	Intrauterine (Laparoscopic)	Least no of sperm	More than themethods listed at 1, 2 & 3	Highest (upto 80%)

Artificial insemination is the main tool for the rapid dissemination of valuable germplasm to improve the genetic quality of farm animals. Though the conception rate with AI is lower but it has great potential to multiply superior quality of goat with faster rate. This technique also spread elite genetic material throughout a population with increased rate of genetic improvement. This technique is also important for breed conservation process and has paved the way for other reproductive biotechnologies. The descript goat population (33%) is very less compared to non-descript and non-productive goats (67%). So, to increase the productivity per goat we need to improve the breed quality scientifically. The sufficient elite germplasm of male buck is not available throughout the country to cover breeding programmed by natural mating. AI is the only solution to improve the quality and productivity per goat.

Freezing of spermatozoa of all the domestic species, is a challenging because of variation in size, shape and lipid composition of sperm from different species. Thus, a cryopreservation protocol for semen of one animal species, may not be necessarily ideal for other. The cryopreservation of goat semen is a complex process that involves balancing of many factors to achieve optimum results. Goat sperm require special attention to maximize the post-thawing viability and fertility. As observed in other domestic animals, the freezing process of semen also reduces the viability of the sperm in goats. In general, around 50-60% of the sperm population survived under cryopreservation with standard protocols. If the total number of fully functional spermatozoa in a cryopreserved semen dose falls below the required number, then fertility would be reduced. The pregnancy rate of 7 to 79% following artificial insemination (AI) with frozen-thawed goat semen has been reported (Bispo et al., 2012).

Artificial Insemination in Goats: An Overview 3 Different researchers reported different fertility rates with cryopreserved goat semen. Factors such as season, breed, and age of the buck and management practices affect the quality and the freezing ability of semen.

Table 2: Pregnancy rate after artificial insemination with frozen-thawed semen in goats

Country	Goat breed	Protocol	Pregnancy rate (%)	Reference
Israel	Saanen	CIDR + equine chorionic gonadotrophin (eCG) Injection	33.90	Gacitua and Arav, 2005
Spain	Florida	FGA Sponge + cloprostenol Injection	42.90	Dorado et al., 2007
	Murciano-Granadina	Progesterone-impregnated sponge+ eCG Injection	55.70	Viudes-de-Castro et al., 2009
	Majorera	FGA Sponge + eCG Injection	42.80	Batista et al., 2009
USA	Anglo-Nubian	-	47.60	Dorado et al., 2007
Norway	Norwegian Dairy	Natural oestrus	57.60	Nordstoga et al., 2010
Argentina	Angora	Natural oestrus	45.50	Gibbons and Cueto, 2011
Bangladesh	Black Bengal	Natural oestrus	43.90	Apu et al., 2012
Bulgaria	Bulgarian White	Natural oestrus	33.30	Yotov et al., 2016
Indonesia	Jawarandu	Natural oestrus	21.00	Nuraini et al., 2021
India	Jamunapari	Natural oestrus	53.12	Kharche et al., 2013
	Non-descript	Natural oestrus	47.00	Ghalsasi and Nimbkar, 2017
	Jamunapari, Barbari	Natural oestrus	37.57	Ranjan et al., 2020

Identification of superior bucks and maximum utilization of their semen for breeding does have been the well-known method for promotion of goat production. Artificial insemination (AI) with freshly diluted buck semen has inherent limitations of rapid loss of sperm motility and consequently and freezing ability, particularly when stored at refrigerated temperature. Obviously largescale propagation of proven buck semen through AI with frozen semen is the only alternative means for increasing the goat productivity. Large scale propagation of buck semen on national as well as international plane is not possible unless a suitable technology for freezing buck semen is developed. The optimum freezing technique and an appropriate semen extender are yet to be successfully achieved.

Future strategies

Critical studies to establish the minimum number of sperm per inseminating dose for acceptable fertility (about 60%) and strict quality control of the frozen semen at various stages of production, processing, storage and final use are necessary. In addition, use of sex-sorted sperm for AI should be promoted as a means of increasing the efficiency of reproduction in goats, especially in the dairy business where males have little commercial value. Sex-sorted semen has been used successfully in several species, including cattle, horses, pigs and sheep but not in goats in India. However, it is expected that this technology can be applied to goat semen. There is need to identify the seminal characteristics which directly affects the freezing ability of spermatozoa. Critical studies to establish the fertility marker-based selection of the bucks for using in semen cryopreservation might be of great importance in years to come.

References

Apu, A. S., Yahia, K. M., Hussain, S. S., Fakruzzaman, M., Notter, D. R. (2012). A comparative study of fresh and frozen-thawed semen quality in relation to fertility of black bengal goats semen from six adult male black bengal goats.

Batista, M., Nino, T., Alamo, D., Castro, N., Santana, M., Gonzalez, F., Gracia, A. (2009). Successful artificial insemination using semen frozen and stored by an ultrafreezer in the Majorera goat breed. *Theriogenology*, *71*(8), 1307-1315.

Bispo, C. A. S., Pugliesi, G., Galvão, P., Rodrigues, M. T., Ker, P. G., Filgueiras, B., Carvalho, G. R. (2011). Effect of low and high egg yolk concentrations in the semen extender for goat semen cryopreservation. *Small Ruminant Research*, *100*(1), 54-58.

Dorado, J., Rodríguez, I., Hidalgo, M. (2007). Cryopreservation of goat spermatozoa: Comparison of two freezing extenders based on post-thaw sperm quality and fertility rates after artificial insemination. *Theriogenology*, *68*(2), 168-177.

Gacitua, H., Arav, A. (2005). Successful pregnancies with directional freezing of large volume buck semen. *Theriogenology*, *63*(3), 931-938.

Ghalsasi, P., Nimbkar, C. (2017). Artificial Insemination in farmers' goats using Osmanabadi breed's frozen semen. In: National Scope on Up-Scaling Production to Products Value Addition and their Safety, ICAR-Central Institute for Research on Goats, Makhdoom, 9-10 November 2017, pp. 71-72.

Gibbons, A., Cueto, M. (2011). Cryopreservation and diffusion of goat genetic material in the Argentine Patagonia. In *Congresso Brasileiro de Reprodução Animal. 19. 2011 05 25-27, 25 al 27 de mayo, 2011. Recife, Brasil. BR.*.

Kharche, S. D., Jindal, S. K., Priyadharsini, R., Kumar, S., Goel, A. K., Ramachandran, N., Rout, P. K. (2013). Fertility following frozen semen artificial insemination in Jamunapari goats. *Indian J. Anim. Sci*, *83*(10), 1071-1073.

Nordstoga, A. B., Söderquist, L., Ådnøy, T., Farstad, W., & Paulenz, H. (2010). Vaginal deposition of frozen-thawed semen in Norwegian dairy goats: comparison of single and double insemination with equal total number of spermatozoa. *Theriogenology*, *74*(5), 895-900.

Nuraini, D. M., Prastowo, S., Widyas, N. (2021). Reproductive performance comparison between natural and artificial service in Jawarandu goat. In *IOP Conference Series: Earth and Environmental Science* (Vol. 637, No. 1, p. 012028). IOP Publishing.

Ranjan, R., Goel, A. K., Kharche, S. D., Priyadharsini, R., Ramachandran, N., Singh, M. K., Chauhan, M. S. (2020). Effect of cervical insemination with frozen semen on fertility of Indian goat breed. *The Indian Journal of Animal Sciences*, *90*(4).

Viudes-de-Castro, M. P., Salvador, I., Marco-Jiménez, F., Gómez, E. A., Silvestre, M. A. (2009). Effect of oxytocin treatment on artificial insemination with frozen–thawed semen in Murciano–Granadina goats. *Reproduction in Domestic Animals*, *44*(4), 576-579.

Yotov, S. A., Velislavova, D. V., Dimova, L. R. (2016). Pregnancy rate in Bulgarian White milk goats with natural and synchronized estrus after artificial insemination by frozen semen during breeding season. *Asian Pacific Journal of Reproduction*, *5*(2), 144-147.

2

Artificial Insemination for Sustainable Goat Production

Ravi Ranjan and Chetna Gangwar

Division of AP&R, ICAR- Central Institute for Research on Goats Makhdoom, Farah-281122, Mathura, Uttar Pradesh

---

The goats play a vital role in the economy of the poor and marginal farmers of rural India. Notwithstanding the fact that the goat population has shown a steady growth over the year's very little effort has been taken for genetic improvement at farm level. As per 20th Livestock Census, 27.74% of the livestock population is Goats. Out of 148.88 million Indigenous Goats (Including Non-descript), 27.4% are pure breed, 9.1% are graded breeds and the remaining 63.5% are non-descript breeds. So, to increase the productivity per goat, we need to improve the breed quality scientifically. Artificial insemination (AI) using frozen semen is practiced to produce superior progeny and to accelerate the up gradation of stock. The conception rate with AI is lower but it has great potential to multiply superior quality of goat with faster rate. This technique also spread elite genetic material throughout a population with increased rate of genetic improvement. This technique is also important for the breed conservation process and has paved the way for other reproductive biotechnologies. The sufficient elite germplasm of male buck is not available throughout the country to cover breeding programmed by natural mating. AI is the best solution to improve the quality and productivity per goat.

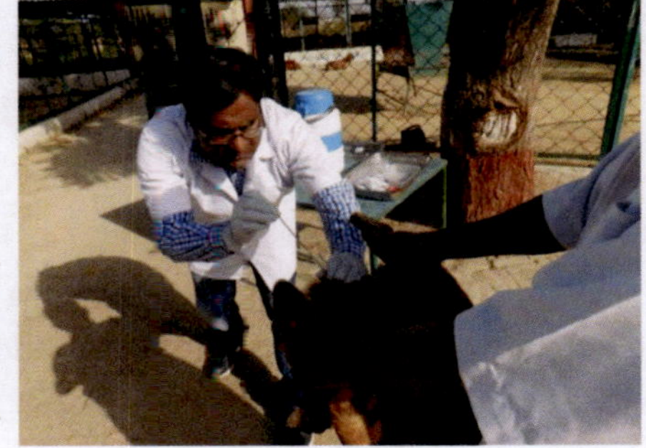

Identification of superior bucks and maximum utilization of their semen for breeding have been considered the well- known method for promotion of goatproduction. Artificial insemination (AI) with freshly diluted buck semen has inherent limitations of rapid lossof sperm motility and consequently freezing ability, particularly when stored at refrigerated temperature.

Obviously large-scale propagation of proven buck semen through AI with frozen semen is the only alternative means for increasing the goat productivity. Large scale propagation of buck semen of national as well as international standard is not possible unless a suitable technology for freezing buck semen is developed. The optimum freezing technique and an appropriate semen extender are yet to be successfully achieved. It would be prudent to have production of quality frozen semen and made it available for its use at large scale. The post-thaw motility and the associated fertility of cryopreserved sperm are found to be reduced in goats due to inappropriate semen extender. The detail molecular mechanism and extent of cryopreservation-associated structural damages to sperm have not been explored systematically. The most potent contributing element identified is the cryopreservation-associated oxidative membrane, protein and DNA damages of sperm.

Table 1. How AI will be helpful

Total goat in the country	148.88 million	
Breedable doe	85 million	
Breedable buck	15 million	
	Natural Mating	AI with frozen semen
One buck cover goat in a year	50	2000
Buck required to cover breedable goat	2 million	50000

Fertility of frozen-thawed semen

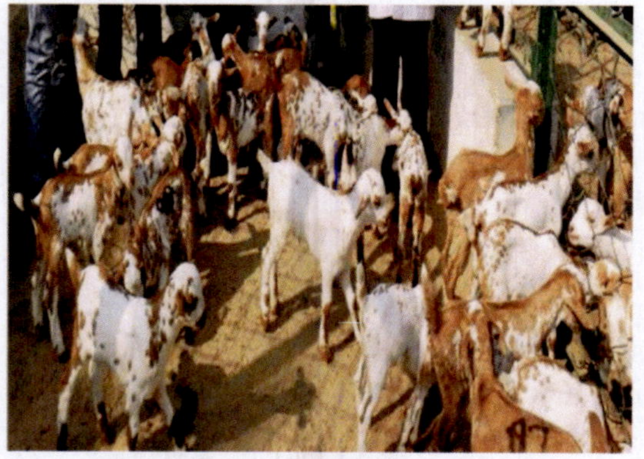

The conception rate achieved at ICAR-CIRG, Mathura with frozen thawed goat semen was 38.5% on actual kidding basis. (Ranjan et al., 2017; Ranjan et al., 2020). ICAR-CSWRI, Avikanagar after trans cervical AI (TCAI) with frozen- thawed ram semen was up to 36% (Naqvi et al.,1998) and this result is very inconsistent which may vary from 0 to 40%. However, much higher conception rate was achieved when frozen-thawed semen is deposited directly in to the uterus through laparoscopy (76%, based on ultrasonography, unpublished data).

Motility and other sperm functions

The average post-thaw motility of cryo-preserved buck semen achieved at ICAR-CIRG, Mathura generally ranged between 45-55% by use of native breeds (Ranjan et al. 2014, 2015). The protocol involving programmable cryo-freezer and using ejaculates having high density (>3x10^9sperm ml^{-1}), rapid wave motion, >70 % initial motility and packaged in French mini strawsresulted in the above motility consistently.

The pioneering work on technique in the goat was carried out at Indian Veterinary Research Institute, Izatnagar (Guha et al., 1951) and Veterinary College, Mathura (Roy and Gupta, 1959: Roy et al. 1962) revealed around 50% conceptions after first insemination with washed spermatozoa diluted in EYC diluents. Though the attempts of AI in goats have been undergoing on experimental basis at various organized farms and Research Institutions of India, still serious and coordinated efforts are lacking for taking up the AI in goats on a large scale like in cattle and buffaloes. Cryopreserved semen is also the hope for restoration of dead valuable bulls through cloning using donor somatic cells isolated from cryopreserved semen (Selokar et al. 2014). Initial work was carried out at National Dairy Research Institute, Chauhan et al. 1997, who found that heparin increased capacitation of buffalo sperm confirmed byelectron microscopy and *in vitro* fertilization. They ruled out the harmful effect of egg yolk on goat semen freezability and advocate egg yolk may be used as a effective freezability increasing extender for goat semen freezing (Chauhan and Anand, 1991). There was also acrosome damage and enzyme leakage of goat spermatozoa during dilution, cooling and freezing (Chauhan et al. 1994). The pioneer work of Sahni and Roy (1972)on deep freezing of buck semen using original Cambridge method (-79^{0}C) revealed 30-40% post thaw motility in citrate yolk and milk diluents containing 3-6% glycerol as cryo-protectant. Later on in 1972, 35-50% survival in buck semen frozen by straw method (-196^{0}C) was observed. Research work on freezability of buck semen with the use of citrate-yolk milkand tris-citrate acid yolk diluents was carried at veterinary colleges of Anand, Guwahati, Tirupati, Ranchi, Bombay, Akola, NARI and Mathura including Central Institute for Research on Goat, irrespective of glycerol percentage (3-9%) and equilibration time (0-6 hrs), post-thaw motility varied between 42-66 percent. Bhattacharyya et al (2012) reported 71.43% pregnancy rate with kidding rate of 1.27 by pellet semen. Conception rate was poor (35-45%) due to deposition of frozen semen over the opening of the cervix. Improvement in fertility (55-65%) was observed due to deep cervical insemination technique (Deka and Rao, 1989; Deshpande and Mehta, 1991). Human population will reach 1.7 billion in India and goat population will be 216 million by 2050 (Vision 2050, ICAR-CIRG). So, to fulfil the requirement in terms of milk, meat and manure to a vast human population, we need to increase the productivity per goat. To cover 71 million breedable does, we need 1.5-2 million bucks as compared to only 50,000 bucks needed for Frozen Semen AI Technology. AI may play a pivotal role for the long-term *ex-situ in-vitro* conservation of threatened breeds *viz.* Jamunapari, Jakhrana, Surti, Beetal, Sangamneri etc. The increase in productivity and performance of large number of non-descriptand low potential goats (>100 million) could be easily upgraded and improvedonly through AI.

AI Procedure and Achievements Methods of AI

1. Intravaginal
2. Intracervical
3. Intrauterine

Intravaginal and Intracervical AI is mainly used by most of workers. Intrauterine method is used for research purpose. There is complex cervical anatomy in goats having 3-6 cartilaginous cervical folds and are horizontally aligned. It is very difficult to pass the AI gun throughout the cervix. So, the conception rate highly correlated with depth of penetration. This technique is more suited in goats and easy to perform. The total time taken is 2-3 minutes. The pregnancy rate is 20-55% (FAO, 2012).

Intra-cervical AI is mainly used to get maximum benefits. For Intra cervical AI, the estrous goat lifted from back for clear visualization of genitalia. A lubricated glass vaginal speculum is inserted through vagina for visualization of cervical opening under sunlight. Then frozen thawed semen straw inserted through vaginal speculum and go through cervical opening and semen was deposited there and waits for two to three minutes.

As per ICAR-CIRG protocol, the post thaw motility in Jamunapari, Barbari, Jakhrana and Sirohi breeds were 52.8±3.54%, 54.4±2.84%, 48.8±3.12% and 46.2±2.32%, respectively. More than 300 kids were born through AI last two years. The success rate (kidding%) during 2018-19 is recorded as 37.74 % which is highest till date (Ranjan et al., 2020a), Fig. 1.

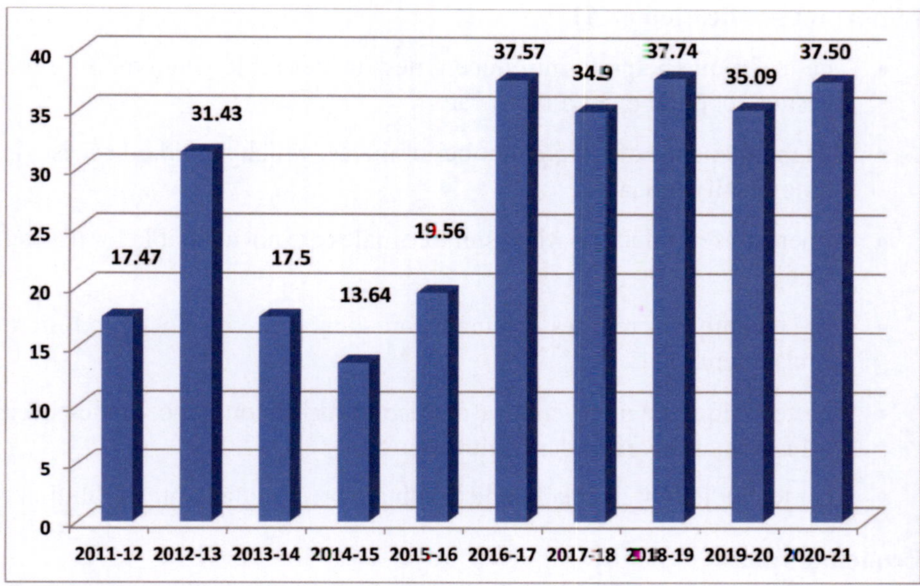

Fig. 1. Kidding % through Artificial Insemination *Source*: ICAR-CIRG

Laparoscopic insemination

Laparoscopic insemination entails elaborate equipment and special skills. Laparoscopic artificial insemination (LAI) with frozen semen yields higher pregnancy rates and allows a reduction in the concentration of the seminal dose (200 vs. 100 million spermatozoa/inseminated goats with the CAI and LAI techniques, respectively). Gibbons et al., 1997 obtained 69% pregnancy rate by LAI with 100 million frozen spermatozoa/insemination dose under optimal conditions in Angora herd. Similarly, other authors with different breeds (Cashmere: Ritar et al., 1990; dairy goats Vallet et al., 1992) reported 20% increase in pregnancy rates when applying LAI in relation to average values of CAI. Pregnancy rates achieved with laparoscopic insemination are approximately 60-80% (Cseh et al, 2012), making use of this technique an attractive option for producers with large numbers of animals requiring insemination. Pregnancy rates of 56.67 % were observed with frozen thawed semen through laparascopic insemination (Anakkul et al. 2014). In concurrence to these findings, Ritar et al. (1990) reported 52.1% pregnancy rates in Cashmere goats and Gibbon et al. (2011) reported 54% pregnancy rates in Angora goats with frozen semen through laparoscopic insemination.

Important application of AI

- The technique helps to introduce a new or desirable genotype into the livestock population at a faster rate.
- The maintenance of a large number of males, which would otherwise, is economically unviable.
- Al permits reproduction when suitable males are not available for natural mating.
- The technique provides accurate breeding records for good herd management.
- The technique helps to control disease transmission, since males used for insemination are under health control.
- This technology will check indiscriminate breeding and breed dilution.

Economic value

Economic value of AI in goat farming, especially by small and marginal farmers, has hardly been realized. It is a cost-effective technique and multiply highquality animals at the faster rate. The extra cost incurred on maintenance of bucks @Rs. 6000/- per annum, can be saved by using AI technique. This will help goat keepers of India to double their income in a short period.

References

Chauhan MS, Anand SR. (1990). Effect of egg yolk lipids on the freezing of goat semen. Theriogenology. 34(5):1003-13.

Chauhan MS, Anand SR. (1991). In vitro maturation and fertilization of goat oocytes. Indian Journal Exp Biol. 29(2):105-10.

Chauhan MS, Kapila R, Gandhi KK, Anand SR. (1994). Acrosome damage and enzyme leakage of goat spermatozoa during dilution, cooling and freezing. Andrologia. 26(1):21-6.

Chauhan MS, Singla SK, Manik RS, Madan ML. (1997). Increased capacitation of buffalo sperm by heparin as confirmed by electron microscopy and in vitro fertilization. Indian Journal Exp Biol. 35(10):1038-43.

Chetna Gangwar, R Ranjan, Satish Kumar, S D Kharche, A K Goel, N Ramachandran and SK Jindal. (2014). Use of chelating agent for optimum post thaw quality of buck semen. Indian Journal of Animal Sciences 84 (8): 839–841.

Hancock J L. (1951). A staining technique for the study of temperature shock in semen. Nature (London). 167: 323.

Kharche, S.D., S.K.Jindal, R. Priyadhrashini, Satish Kumar, A.K.Goel, N. Ramachandran and Rout, P.K. (2013) Fertility following frozen semen artificial insemination in Jamunapari goats. Indian Journal of Animal Sciences 83(10) 1071-1073.

Priyadharsini, R., Jindal, S.K., Sharma, D., Ramachandran, N., Kharche, S.D. and Goel, A.K. 2011. Effect of Different Egg Yolk Level on the Cryopreservation Capability of Jakhrana Goat Semen. Journal of Animal Science Advances 1(1):28-37.

Ranjan R, Goel A K, Kharche S D, Ramachandran N, Gangwar Chetna and Jindal S K. (2014). Comparison between normal and dual staining technique for evaluating acrosome status and viability in frozen thawed buck spermatozoa. The Indian Journal of Small Ruminants 20(2): 50-53.

Ranjan R, Goel A.K, N. Ramachandran, S.D. Kharche and S.K. Jindal. (2015). Effect of egg yolk levels and equilibration periods on freezability of Jamunapari buck semen. The Indian Journal of Small Ruminants 21(1): 32-36.

Ranjan R, Ramachandran N, Jindal S K and Sinha N K. 2009b. Hypo osmotic swelling test in frozen thawed goat spermatozoa. Indian Journal of Animal Science 79 (10):1022-1023.

Ranjan R, Ramachandran, Jindal S K, Sinha N K, Goel A K, S D Kharche and Sikarwar A K S. 2009a. Effect of egg yolk levels on keeping quality of Marawari buck semen at refrigeration temperature. Indian Journal of Animal Science 79 (7):10-13.

Saraswat Sonia, Jindal S K, Kharche S D, Rout P K, Ranjan R and Priyadharsini R. 2014. Roleof antioxidant additives in the protection of DNA integrity of buck spermatozoa with RAPD assay. Indian Journal of Animal Sciences 84 (3): 295–297.

Selokar NL, Saini M, Palta P, Chauhan MS, Manik R, Singla SK. (2014). Hope for restorationof dead valuable bulls through cloning using donor somatic cells isolated from cryopreserved semen. PLoS One. 10;9 (3):e90755.

Watson P F. (1975). Use of Giemsa stain to detect changes in acrosomes of frozen ram spermatozoa. Veterinary Records 97:12–15.

3

Anatomy of Buck Genital System

Shriprakash Singh, M.M. Farooqui, Abhinov Verma and Chanda Singh

Department of Anatomy, College of Veterinary Science and Animal Husbandry, DUVASU, Mathura-281 001, Uttar Pradesh

The male genital system consists of:

1. The pair gonads, the testes
2. Epididymis
3. Vas deference or ductus deference
4. Accessory glands (Seminal vesicles, prostate glands, & bulbo-urethral glands)

Testes

The testes of buck are the primary sex organ and oval in shape, paired with two borders (anterior and posterior), two surfaces (medial and lateral) and two extremities (proximal and distal). The left testis is heavier, longer and thicker than the right. The testes of buck are broader in proportion to their length. They are symmetrical in shape and size, elastic to firm in consistency, and mobile in the scrotal sac. A buck within 8-14 months of age should have 25 cm of scrotal circumference. The testis is covered by a cutaneous pouch the scrotum. They lie in the inguinal region, with their longitudinal axis in a vertical position for the bull, buffalo, ram and buck, but divers in the stallion that their axis are in a horizontal position. For camel, the testes are located in the perineal region just under the anus, with their longitudinal axis in an oblique position. The testes are suspended by the spermatic cord. The lateral surface is convex and smooth while the medial surface is flattened owing to its contact with septum scroti. The cranial border is convex while the caudal border is straight to which epididymis is attached. Dorsal and ventral extremities are blunt and rounded. The mean weight of testis in buck range from 132 to 160gms. Each testis is covered by a fibrous tunic named as tunica albuginea. The testes are protected by many layers of tunics *viz.* the tunica vaginalis – parietal and visceral layers which are brought by the testis during its descents. Beside this spermatic fascia and skin and the tunica dartos also protect the testis. During the descent of testis, a peritoneal fold detached from the caudal end of gonad and extended up to abdominal floor on 42nd days known as gubernaculums. During the descent, the testis displaced through the metanephros, abdominal cavity, inguinal region and finally descent into scrotum. In goat, the nephric displacement is completed on 60th day of intrauterine life. The abdominal migration is reached on 80th day of intrauterine life. The testis is situated in theinguinal canal between 89 to 95 days of intrauterine life. The scrotal migration is achieved by 96th day onwards of intrauterine life but process of complete descent of testis in scrotum occurs after birth. The descent of testis from the genital ridge in the foetal to extra corporeal location after birth is mandatory development process to ensure that the mature testis normal spermatogenesis.The gubernaculums testis seems to be most important structure involved in testicular migration. The role of the gubernaculums in testicular migration is especially due to its ability to dilate and shorten, thus facilitating the testis course through the inguinal canal. The testicular descent occurs in mid gestationfor the bull, buffalo, ram and buck and just before or after birth for the stallion, camel, dog and tom cat (2-5 days after birth). Weights of testis are about 100-150grams. The size diverts according to deferent species. The largest testis weight is for the bull (300-400g), followed by the ram (250-300g), buffalo (200-300g), stallion (150-250g) buck (100-150g), and camel (60-100g). In mature bucks, they may change in size during the breeding season. In the case of rams and bucks' testes there are seasonal variations in spermatogenic activity with the greatest activity occurring in autumn. The testes are cytogenicas well as steroidogenic gland which produces the spermatozoa, the male sex cells and the male sex hormone i.e. testosterone.

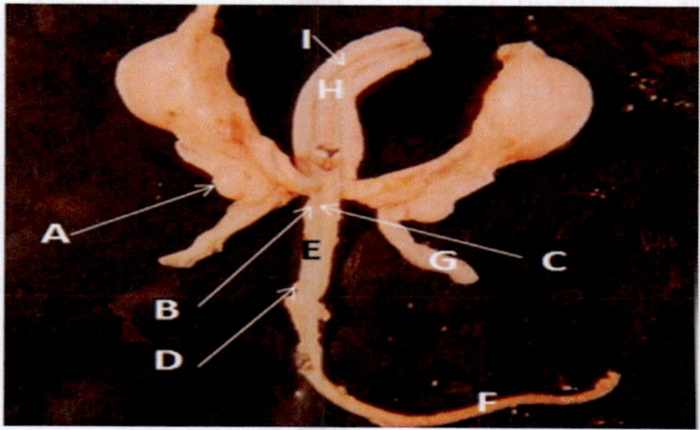

Fig. 1: Male genital System of 100 days old buck foetus. **A**- Left & Right Testis, **B**- Seminal vesicles, **C**- Interglandular groove **D**- Bulbourethral Gland, **E**- Pelvic Urethra, **F**- Penis, **G**- gubernaculum, H- Bladder

Spermatic Cord

The spermatic cords are very long making the testis pendulous during the walk. It consists of spermatic arteries, spermatic veins, internal spermatic nerve, lymphatic, internal cremaster muscles, vas difference and tunica vaginalis visceral layer. Tunica vaginalis is an out pocketing of parietal peritoneum passing through the inguinal canal into the scrotum. It is flask shaped and has narrow proximal part and dilated distal part. The proximal part contains the spermatic cord and distal part has testis and epididymis. The parietal layers lines scrotum and inguinal canal and are continuous with the parietal layer of peritoneum at abdominal inguinal ring. The visceral layer covers the spermatic cord, testis and epididymis. A capillary space is present between parietal and visceral layer which contain a small serous fluid. The spermatic arteries, vein, nerve and lymphatic forms the cranial part of the cord. These are united by connective tissues, interspersed with the internal cremaster muscles. The caudo-medial part of the cord formed by ductus deferens, enclosed in a separate fold of tunica vaginalis. Spermatic cord of buck is very long as compare to other domestic animals. It is a complex structure subjected to various surgical intervention and techniques used for castration, cryptorchidism and inguinal hernia etc.

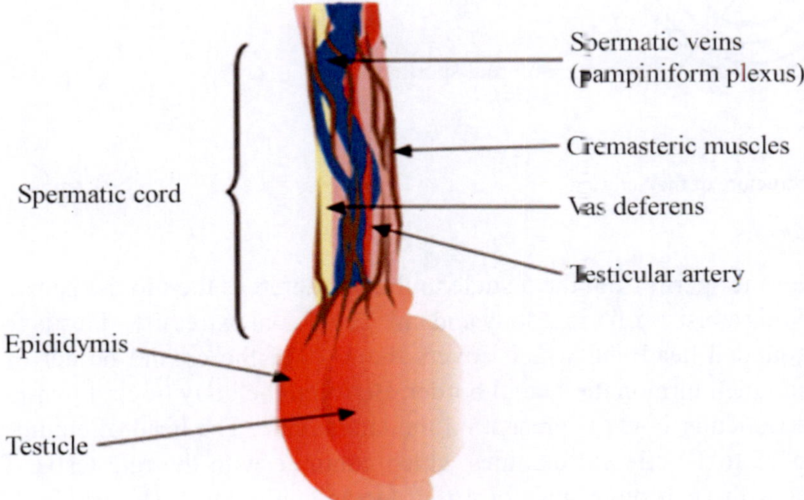

Fig. 2: Showing structure of the spermatic cord

Scrotum

The scrotum is a pouch-like two-lobed sac that encloses the testes and is found hanging below between the two legs of the buck in the inguinal region. The wall of the scrotum is composed of four layers; skin, tunica dartos muscle, scrotal fascia and parietal layer of vaginal tunic. The tunica dartos forms the median septum which divides the scrotum into two distinct pouches. Improper scrotal function and poor testicular distention during hot weather may lead to temporary infertility in bucks. The scrotum is responsible for thermoregulation; provide the favorable environment by powering temperature to produce spermatozoa.

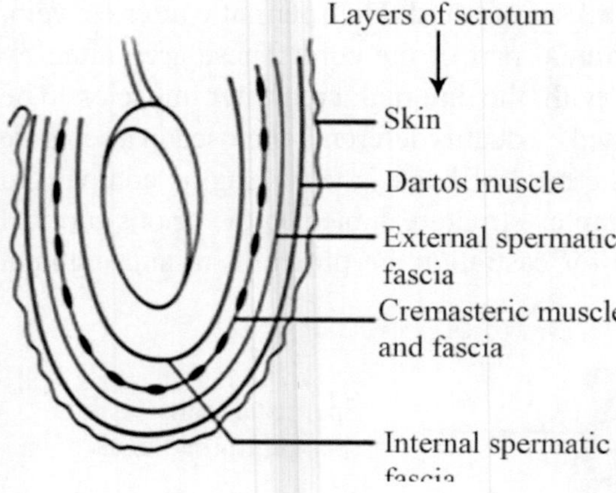

Fig. 3: Structure of the Scrotum

Epididymis

It carries the sperm from the testicle to the vas deferens then to the penis. The epididymis consists of head, body and tail. The dorsal extremity of testis forms a flat rounded head and which covers the 1/4th of the cranial border of the testis and then turn on the lateral border. Between the body of epididymis and testis a testicular bursa is present on the lateral side. The head of epididymis contain 15 to 19 efferent ductules which continue with the rate testis. They connect with each other and form the ductus epididymis. The cauda of the epididymis is rounded and elongated. The head of epididymis is spread on the dorsal extremity of the testis. Length of epididymal tube in buck is about 50m. The left epididymis is longer than right. Sperm continue to develop (mature) in the epididymis and are stored there. The epididymis plays an important role in maturation, storage and transportation of spermatozoa.

Vas deferens

It is a slender, muscular tube that runs from the tail of the epididymis to the neck of the bladder, where it joins the ampulla and accessory sex glands. It is very tortuous in its initial course which passes along the caudal border of the testis. Then it becomes straight in caudal border of spermatic cord and passes through the inguinal canal. It deviates from other structures at the vaginal ring and turns backward into the pelvic cavity. The duct passes backward towards the dorsal surface of bladder and reaches to the caudal part of bladder. The ducts from both the side open at the roof of beginning of pelvic urethra as a slit like opening, the ejaculatory orifice on either side of colliculus seminalis. After crossing the ureter in the abdominal cavity it dilates into a spindle shaped enlargement, the ampulla The epithelium of ampulla thrown into numerous thin irregularly branching folds which show evidence of secretion. Primary function is to move sperm into the urethra at the time of ejaculation. In vasectomised animals (teaser bucks) the animal still produces testosterone and sperm cells. The vas deferens is the tubular structure which conducts the spermatozoa to the urethra.

Accessory sex glands

The male accessory sex glands include vesicular glands or seminal vesicle, prostate gland and bulbourethral or cowpers gland. They secrete fluids into urethra during ejaculation. These fluids contain sugars to nourish the sperm, buffers to prevent rapid changes in pH and other chemicals that serve to protect and propel the sperm out of the urethra and into the vagina.

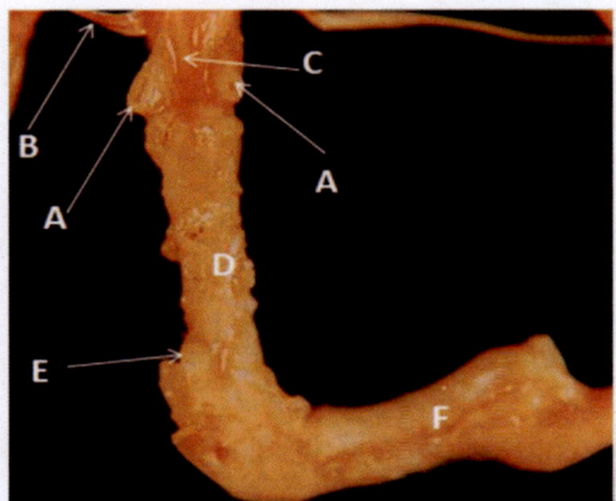

Fig. 4: Accessory sex glands of buck

A. Seminal vesicles **B.** vas deference **C.** ampulla **D.** pelvic urethra **E.** bulbo urethral gland **F.** Body of penis

Seminal vesicles

They are two compact lobulated glands located on dorsolateral aspect of neck of the urinary bladder. The execratory ducts open on either side of coliculus seminalis lateral to opening of vas deferens. Each gland 3 to 4 cms long in length. The duct of the seminal vesicles and the ductus deferens may share a common ejaculatory duct that opens into the urethra. They are pair of compact lobular glands that are easily identified because of their knobby appearance in the buck. In the stallion, they are large pyriform glandular sac that evades identification because of their thin wall. In the stallion and boar, the seminal vesicles are sac-like, but in the buck the vesicles are lobulated and firmer. The vesicular glands are lobulated gland identified because of their appearance like cluster of grapes.

Prostate Gland

Prostate gland is a single fibero-muscular-glandular structure with 2 parts, a body that stretches across the dorsal surface of the neck of the urinary bladder and disseminate or internal part that surrounds the pelvic urethra. The body of theprostate is small in the bull and large in the boar and camel, but absent in the ram and buck. The prostate gland in the stallion is bilobed and wholly external that can be identified by palpation per rectum. The prostatic duct opens in pelvic urethra behind the colicullus seminalis. Each gland is covered by urethral muscles which is thin dorsally and ventrally and thick laterally. Prostate gland hasa major contribution in the seminal fluid which plays important role in male fertility. It neutralizes the seminal plasma and to initiate active movement of ejaculated spermatozoa. The prostatic secretion is rich in various enzymes.

Bulbourethral Gland

They are paired rounded or ovoid in shape. Each gland is located on either side of pelvic urethra at the level of ischial arch and is covered by distinct fibrous capsule having thick bundles of striated bulbocavernosus muscles. Each gland has single duct opens in urethra behind the duct of prostate. The bulbourethral gland or Cowper's gland of the buck, stallion, bull and ram are small, round structures lying between the anus and the urethra. Normal seminal volume during ejaculation for a buck is 0.5-1.5 ml, with a concentration of 1.5-6.0 billion sperm cells/ml. The bulbourethral glands add fluids to semen during the process of ejaculation, which act as lubricant and make the semen less watery to provide a suitable living environment for sperm.

Urethra Bucks possess a structure called a filiform appendage which is extension of the urethra beyond the end of the penis. The urethra is the duct which carries urine or sperm out of the buck's body. Urethra consists of two parts:

1. Pelvic Urethra
2. Penile Urethra

Pelvic Urethra – The pelvic urethra is a complex muscular tube, which extends from urinary bladder to the ischial arch and it is a common passage for both urinary and reproductive system. All the three accessory sex glands pour their secretion to the urethra. It lies on the floor of pelvic cavity and surrounded by the urethral muscle. The lumen is narrow at the level of ischial arch then it is continued as penile urethra.

Penile Urethra – It passes between two crura of penis and turns forward and included in the body of penis. It contains corpus cavernosus and bulbo cavernosus muscles. The urethra lies in the grooves on ventral surface of corpus cavernosum penis. The terminal portion of penile urethra protrude 1.5 inch beyond the glans penis is known as process urethrae. The opening from the urinary bladder into the urethra is known as internal urethral orifice and terminal opening of urethra is known as external urethral orifice.

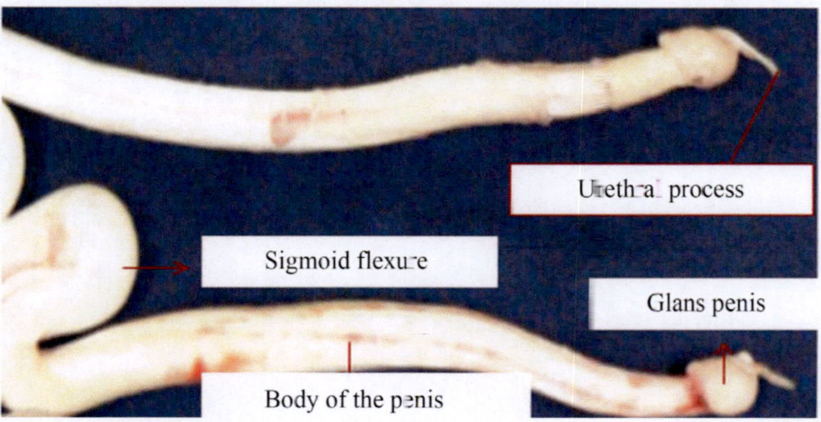

Fig. 5: Penis and urethra of the Buck

Penis – It is male copulatory organ composed of fibrous and erectile tissue (fibro elastic nature). The penis is fibro-elastic (with sigmoid flexure) in buck, bull and camel but vascular, musclo cavernosus and hemodynamic in the stallion. The average length of the penis is about 40 cm. It contains root, body and glans. The root is attached to lateral part of ischial arch by two crura and between them bulbus penis is present. The crura are covered by two symmetrical muscles that act in erection of penis. The bulbus penis is posterior expansion of corpus spongiosum penis which is erectile tissue of penis. The body begins at the junction of two crura. It consists of paired corpus cavernosum penis and the penile urethra is surrounded by corpus spongiosum penis. At origin it is attached to symphysis ischia by two strong bands suspensory ligaments of penis. Just behind the scrotum it forms 'S' shape sigmoid flexure. The sigmoid flexure is post-scrotal for the bull and buck, but pre-scrotal for the camel and boar. Vascular erection is not a very prominent feature of erection. The main factor, which increases the length of the penis during erection, is the obliteration of the sigmoid flexure of the organ. In the non-erect state, the glans of the penis is contained in the sheath. The ram and buck have urethral process known as a filiform appendage extending beyond the glans penis. The end of the buck penis is coiled, especially during copulation. Mating time is very short in bucks. Intromission usually lasts less than 5 seconds. Bucks will generally throw their head back at ejaculation.

Glans Penis – It is the free end of penis. The prepuce is very short and tubular sheet covering the cranial free portion of penis in non-erectile state.

4

Physiology of Buck Reproduction

Vikas Sachan[1] and Chetna Gangwar[2]

[1]Department of Veterinary Gynaecology and Obstetrics DUVASU Mathura-281001, Uttar Pradesh
[2]Animal Physiology and Reproduction Division, ICAR- Central Institute for Research on Goats, Makhdoom, Mathura, Uttar Pradesh

- In male animals, endocrine regulation of reproduction is mainly controlled by pituitary gonadotrophins and gonadal androgens. It is not same as in females as there is only negative feedback controls in case of male while it is positively as well as negatively feedback control in females. In other words the synchrony of pituitary gonadotrophins with gonads in male is non cyclic while in female it is cyclic i.e. after castration the pulse frequency of LH and FSH is retained

- Sex Hormones are sex specific e.g. estrogen and progesterone works primarily in females and testosterone in males but sex specificity is limited as far as sexual behaviour is concern. As estrogen injection in castrated buck recovers the maleness while testosterone injection in ovariectomized female maintain the receptivity for male up to certain extent.

- Hypothalamus acts as interface between nervous system and endocrine system. GnRH synthesized in neurons in hypothalamus, released at nerve endings episodic manner and transferred via hypophyseal portal system to anterior pituitary to stimulate the secretion of gonadotrophins.

- Male reproduction is mainly controlled by androgens (Testosterone) secreted by gonads or teticles under the influence of pituitary gonadotrophins (LH and FSH). Pituitary gonadotrophins are synthesized and secreted in response to the hypothalamic gonadotrophin releasing hormones (GnRH).

- Growth hormone, insulin and insulin-like growth factor (IGF)-1 have stimulatory effect on the action of LH over LH receptors.

- LH receptors are found on the leydig cells and on germ cells. Testosterone receptors are found on the leydig cells, sertoli cells and myoid cells but not on the germ cells.
- LH receptors are less in no. and less sensitive on leydig cells up to the age of 6-7 months of age i.e. up to this age LH secretion does not stimulate the secretion or rise in the level of testosterone. Growth hormone, insulin and insulin-like growth factor (IGF)-1 have stimulatory effect on the action of LH over LH receptors.
- Acting on the leydig cells, LH regulates steroidogenesis. LH controls the transformation of cholesterol into pregnenolone (rate-limiting step of testosterone steroidogenesis). Pregnenolone converts into progesterone and further into testosterone (18 °C) in leydig cells.
- LH (lutenizing hormone) is secreted in a pulsatile fashion. Episodes of LH secretion from anterior pituitary occur after each 2-4 hr under the influence of hypothalamic GnRH (4-10 peaks of LH per day). LH acts through LH receptors found on the leydig cells and leads to testosterone synthesis. After 30-60 minutes of LH pulse the level of testosterone is at peak which becomes basal again after 40-80 minutes. The increased level of testosterone imposes negative feedback over hypothalamus as well as pituitary.
- Synthesized androgen (testosterone) converts into DHT (5α-dihydrotestosterone) in sertoli cells and accessory sex glands by 5α-reductase enzyme. Testosterone converts into estradiol in sertoli cells by aromatase enzyme. High level of blood estrogen is an indicative of sertoli cell tumor and occurs mainly in canines.
- There is negative feedback response of both of these products (DHT and estradiol) at the level of hypothalamus and pituitary for LH secretion.
- DHT is more potent androgen than testosterone as DHT does not undergo aromtization. DHT mailnly controls accessory sex gland activity whereas testosterone is the primary androgen involved in spermatogenesis. Both testosterone and DHT bound by androgen-binding protein (ABP) within the reproductive tract lumen and maintain high androgen concentrations in the seminiferous tubules and epididymis.
- Maximum testosterone is transported in the blood in bound form with α-globulin and some form is free which is converted into DHT.
- FSH (follicle stimulating hormone) is secreted in non episodic pattern. FSH regulates the proliferation of sertoli cells in prepubertal life

i.e. determine the sertoli cell numbers at puberty. It determines the postpubertal spermatogenic yield as sertoli cells regulate the process of spermatogenesis.

- The functions of sertoli cell are under control of FSH. Under control of FSH, sertoli cells secrete:

1. Androgen binding protein (ABP) – It binds the androgen (testosterone and DHT) and maintain their concentration in seminiferous tubules and epididymis. Steroid binding protein in males is α-globulin.
2. Activin – It regulates the development of leydig cells in fetal testes and at puberty. It is also responsible for the delay in growth of leydig cells till puberty. It promotes the secretion of FSH at pituitary level.
3. Inhibin – It regulate the various differentiating and growth factor functions. It regulates leydig cell function also. It also exerts negative feedback effect on the secretion of FSH at pituitary level. Inhibin B is more potent and predominant in most of the species whereas in Ram, inhibin A is found to be more potent.
4. Anti-mullerian hormone or Mullerian inhibiting hormone (MIH) – It inhibits the development and differentiation of mullerian duct system or paramesonephric duct system in embryonic life i.e. responsible for the development of male fetus.
5. Transferrin – Source of iron for sperm.
6. Glutathion – Acts as anti-oxidant
7. Insulin like growth factor

- Sertoli cells are also known as nursing mother cells or sustentacular cells. They regulate spermatogenesis and nourish the spermatozooas.
- Prolactin receptors are present on leydig cells. This hormone promotes the functions of LH receptor on leydig cells. But high level of prolactin, growth hormone (GH/STH) and melatonin exerts negative feedback action for production and release of gonadotrophins i.e. responsible for delayed development of sexual characters and sexual behavior (delayed puberty and libido)
- FSH is responsible for the initiation of spermatogenesis but FSH and testosterone both are required for the maintenance of spermatogenesis process and spermiation.

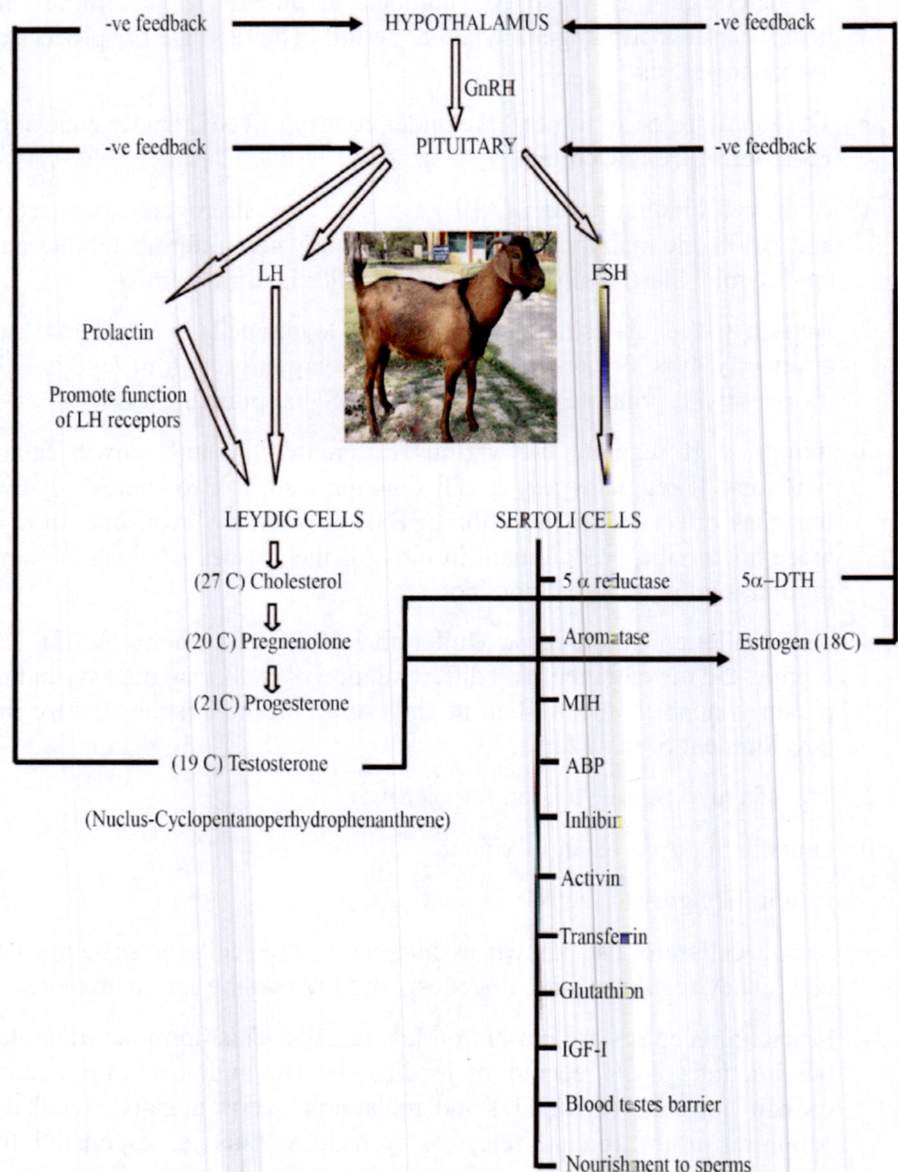

Functions of androgen

1. Testicular descend
2. Sexual differentiation of male reproductive system
3. Regulation of structure and function of accessory sex glands and ductus system

4. Spermatogenesis
5. Development of secondary sexual characters and maleness (Body confirmation, hairs, beard, broad shoulder, aggressiveness, muscle growth etc)
6. Pronlongation of epididymal sperm life
7. Different sexual behavior pattern in different species
8. Penile and prepucial growth. Degeneration of penile frenulum

- Prepubertal castration leads to absence of libido, underdeveloped genitalia and no mating behavior. Post pubertal castration leads to stoppage of ejaculation first then mounting behavior and then penile erection stop.
- Thyroid stimulating hormone (TSH), Growth hormone (STH), Adrenocorticotrophic hormone, Melatonin are necessarily required for maintenance of male reproduction but their over secretion may lead to reverse or negative feedback effect.
- Oxytocin also plays role in increasing tubal activity at the time of ejaculation leads to increased seminal volume with more sperm concentration.
- Some endogenous opioid peptides like β-endorphin present in testicular interstitial fluid in high volume and participate in leydig cell steroidogenesis.
- But ram is more reproductively active during short days. Unlike stallion, due to short day length the increased melatonin secretion reaches to hypothalamus and stimulates the pulsatile secretion of GnRH which in turn responsible for more steroid production. Reducing the day light hours in ram reduce the prolactin production. It leads to increased gonadotrophins secretion and hence testosterone.

5

Selection of Breeding Buck for Improved Production through Artificial Insemination

M.K. Singh, Gopal Dass and Akhilesh Kumar

Division of Animal Genetics, ICAR-CIRG, Makhdoom, Farah-281122 Mathura, Uttar Pradesh

India is the largest goat producing countries in the world exhibiting rich diversity between and within goat breeds. The implementation of a genetic improvement programme requires a clear breed-based breeding objectives and selection criteria, tailored to the needs of goat farming community. Indigenous goat breeds bear a great degree of adaptability for climatic stress, tropical diseases and low quality feed resources, require low inputs for enhancing productivity, thus, little investment along with use of high merit bucks bring a great change in the economy of the farmers. There are currently 37 recognized goat breeds in the country which are kept mostly in small herds on extensive or partial semi-intensive feeding system. Productivity of Indigenous goats, however, observed less than their actual genetic potential and attributed to low input system, lack of suitable breed specific structural genetic improvement programme and poor adoption of technologies. A buck is the most important animal in the herd. A breeding male or buck contributes 50% of the genetic merit of the herd and also determine the future improvement rate. The buck has the greatest genetic impact on the entire herd improvement therefore, should be chosen by taking all cares and measures. However, hardly 30% flocks in India owned buck and mostly of them are of low potency or impure resulting in low or no genetic improvement in the flock. Goat keepers with small flock are not keeping buck primarily due to lack of housing space for buck, expenses on feed and other items on its management and also due to lack of need realization of quality bucks. Lesser availability of purebred and potential bucks is also attributed to sale of good males at early ages (6-12 month) in lieu of little higher prices offered by butcher/buyers and also due to indiscriminate castration by farmers themselves.

Artificial insemination (AI) using frozen semen is highly disseminated reproductive technology in the field of animal breeding and is meaningful only when semen of high genetic merit bucks is utilized. Therefore, establishment of breed wise buck mother farms for the production of high merit bucks and their utilization through artificial insemination is the need of hour. Artificial insemination provides an opportunity to exploit genetic potential of the superior sires. In Indian scenario, a quality buck could be selected based on information from pedigree, individual, progeny and relatives. Multi-stage selection could be the best option for selecting a buck for frozen semen as well herd improvement. Those males which are progeny of purebred parents, progeny of high performing parents, pure-bred as individual healthy, large in size as per age and breed standards (+1 S.D.) should be allowed in ranking (selection process). If data is available on feed conversion efficiency of individual male, then this trait may also be included in selection index. While selecting a buck at progressive farmer level, the candidate male possesses good height, length, weight and conformation (+1 S.D.) i.e., 35 to 40% higher than flock average. Following are phenotype and anatomical attributes of buck selection.

(1) The general appearance of candidate male includes age, health status, conformation, and body condition score. Candidate male should be more masculine (head, neck, heavy shoulder, high bone dimension and more muscles), healthy (disease free), sound footed with proper toe.

(2) Rump and rear leg should be strong for smooth breeding process. Avoid bucks with feet problems such as laminitis and arthritis as it causes pain and adversely affect copulation

(3) Scrotum of bucks should be large as it is positively associated with semen quantity and quality.

(4) Both testicles should be large (well developed) and similar in size, as larger testicles are capable of producing more quantity of sperm cells.

(5) Buck before allowing in selection process may be screened for abnormalities of sexual organs such as testicular atrophy, testicular hypoplasia, testicular degeneration, cryptorchidism, orchitis Once buck is initially selected based on pedigree, phenotype and phenotypic performances, they should be screened for libido, quality sperm or fertilizing and freezing ability.

(6) Buck should be able to transmit its characteristics in its progeny and should not be carrier of any genetic disease.

(7) A buck should dominantly display mating behavior (sexual interest) during breeding and bears a good sense of smell and structural soundness (malformation of the penis and prepuce).

(8) Candidate male should not be obese and a male reared under semi-intensive management may be preferred as buck.

(9) Use of a buck through artificial insemination may also require training of buck for exhibiting sexual behavior and semen collection.

The criteria and methods of buck selection are primarily depending upon purpose of goat farming (milk, meat, fibre). Mass selection (Individual phenotype) is the best for meat (growth) and progeny testing is the best for milk production traits. In Indian context, growth (meat) traits contribute lion share in income therefore, mass selection is the preferred method of selection under which a selection index is constructed and buck are ranked according to their score. Six-month body weight of a kid, 60 days milk yield of their dam and type of birth in small size breeds (Black Bengal), Nine-month body weight of a kid, 90 days milk yield of their dam and type of birth in medium and large size breeds (Barbari, Beetal, Sirohi) constituted the index. The puberty age of male depends on breed (breed size), feeding management and agro-climatic conditions. In general, a male is ready for breeding services at 7-8 month in small size, 9-10 month in medium size and 11-12 month in large size goat breeds. For higher conception, better freezability and long- term utilization, a buck should be utilized after attaining proper physical and physiological maturity. Therefore, right age to start/obtain quality conception/semen is >11 month in small size (Black Bengal, Teressa), >14 month in medium size (Surti, Barbari) and >16 month in large size goat breed (Beetal, Jamunapari, Sirohi).

At field level, kids at 3-6 months of age based on their breed purity, body weight, body size, type of birth, body conditions, built, mother's milk yield could be initially selected twice of requirement. These males again ranked at 9-12 months of age depending upon breed size including physical confirmation, libido, status of reproductive organs-scrotum, testicle (atrophy, hypoplasia), prepuce, penis etc. and semen quality.

The semen quality in terms of quantitative seminal traits like volume, sperm density per ml and per ejaculate and the qualitative traits like color, consistency and mass activity, progressive motility, live sperms (%), abnormal sperms (%) need to be evaluated before using the bucks for mating in the flock. If the values of above parameters are beyond the norms suggested for use, then the individual bucks should not be used for breeding and needs to be culled promptly.

Top rank male on above-described characteristics should be selected, thereafter tested for libido, semen quality and finally for fertility rate. Bucks with better libido and semen qualities in terms of volume, sperm concentration, mass motility etc. are finally selected and use them as breeding bucks. The breeding bucks donated semen from 0.2 to 1.0 ml with creamy & thick consistency and mass motility from +3.0 to +5.0 and found negative in Brucella screening are finally selected and used for breeding. Desspite all precautions some bucks or their semen does not work satisfactory therefore cull them immediately.

Improvement in meat production through selection

The indigenous breeds possess high genetic variability with respect to meat production traits. It can be gainfully exploited through selection. However, proper attempts have not been made so far involving large population and optimum inputs required to express their potential and performance. Pre-slaughter body weight at 6 months of age is the simplest criterion for improving meat production. Although hot carcass weight and dressing percentages have high heritability. These traits cannot be measured in live animals. Therefore, there is a need to assess the correlated responses that can be accrued in carcass traits along with the expected response to selection in the prime trait. It was observed that selection based on 6 months body weight will bring about genetic improvement to a tune of 1.01 kg in the trait itself along with an improvement of 0.531 kg in hot carcass weight as a correlated trait under a selection pressure of one standard deviation above the population mean.

Method of selection

The method of selection is decided on the basis of the nature of inheritance of the traits under selection. For quantitative traits with high heritability, mass selection is the appropriate method. The heritability of body weight traits is moderately high and can be measured in both sexes. Therefore, mass selection based on phenotypic value will improve the trait. But magnitude of improvement will be higher by selecting sires on the basis of their breeding values, computed from the performance of their progeny. The accuracy of progeny testing of course depends upon the environmental condition and the number of progenies evaluated per sire. In a progeny-testing Programme involving 25 bucks and 500 does, the magnitude of genetic gain in weaning weight was 35% higher through progeny-testing over individual selection.

Thus, sire evaluation through progeny testing may be preferred over mass selection for improving meat production at organized farm.

The important Selection criteria should depend upon the phenotypic and genetic variances and co-variances among important characters, their relative economics values and sources of information. The age at first kidding and kidding interval has moderate heritability and litter size pre-weaning survival has low h^2. Body weight, growth rate, carcass yield and quality have reasonably high h^2. Milk yield have medium h^2. For improving meat production, selection on 6 months body weight may be most feasible and bring reasonable genetic progress in meat production through improving reproduction, body weight gain and carcass yield. Superior breeding bucks may be identified in farmers flock through objective assessment of flocks for producing genetically superior males for the improvement in field. Goats of very high genetic merit identified in field and may be transferred to institute flock or Nucleus breeding herd. The best males should be retained in the institutional flock for breeding with elite females for producing males and rest be made available to the flock owners.

Selection in open nucleus flocks: For more efficient selection programme, involvement of farmers into co-operative breeding schemes is essential. Keeping nucleus flock open would help in breeding and increasing selection intensity through continuous introduction of superior animals from the farmer's flocks. After distribution of the males to the cooperative flocks, rest could be distributed to the other flocks to be improved. Subsequently, flocks of co-operating farmers could also be utilized in breeding males through selection of males from the nucleus (multiplier flocks). Such selection scheme will bring faster genetic progress.

6

Breeding Soundness Evaluation through Ultrasonography of Buck Testes

Chetna Gangwar and S.D. Kharche

Division of AP&R, ICAR- Central Institute for Research on Goats Makhdoom, Farah-281122, Mathura, Uttar Pradesh

Ultrasonography

Ian Donald in the year **1956** used the one-dimensional A-mode (amplitude mode) to measure the parietal diameter of the fetal head and thus introduced the ultrasound in diagnostic and medicine. Ultrasonography does not use radiation or powerful magnetic field as source of energy and the equipment cost is usually affordable. This modality involves the use of sound waves in viewing the longitudinal, sagittal and transverse planes for both testes . Sound is measured in cycles per second or hertz (Hz); the audible range of sound is from 20-20,000 Hz. Diagnostic ultrasound is usually in the range of 1–20 megahertz (MHz).

The speed of sound depends on the tissues through which it propagates because density and compressibility change the speed, the sound wave travels. On an average the assumed speed of sound in soft tissue is 1540 m/s.

Transducer

A transducer or probe consists of a cable connecting it to the ultrasound machine, a plastic casing which encloses the electronics, a damping material, piezoelectric crystals, a matching layer and a protective layer. It is designed to convert an electronic pulse into an ultrasound pulse, then convert the sound pulse into an electronic signal in order to be processed to produce an image.

Each Piezoelectric crystal is electronically and acoustically isolated from all the others, so each crystal transmits its own individual ultrasound wave, these waves join together to form a single wavefront. By timing the firing of the crystals, we can steer the beam, or focus the beam at multiple levels.

The part of the transducer which is in contact with the patient is called the face of the transducer, and the shape and size of this face is termed the '**footprint**'. The face of the transducer has different shapes.

A Linear array transducer has all the piezoelectric crystals set in a line across the transducer face. This produces a rectangular ultrasound image and is usually used for:

- Vessels
- Vascular access
- Needle guidance
- Musculoskeletal imaging
- Small parts such thyroid
- Foreign bodies
- Anywhere we need a wide 'near field' but not a lot of depth. Linear transducers tend to be higher in frequency than curved arrays.

A curved array transducer is a transducer where the crystals are arranged along a curved surface, to produce a wide near field, and a wide far field. The image produced has a curved upper and lower edge. This type of transducer is usually used for:

- Abdominal
- Obstetric
- Anywhere we need a lower frequency and good depth penetration
- Where difficult or deep vessels in abdomen need to be seen

A phased array transducer, is one in which the crystals are fired in phases to produce a pizza slice shaped image on the monitor. This transducer may also be called a "Sector Transducer". This type of transducer is usually used for:

- Cardiac imaging and
- Difficult or deep intercostal views of the abdomen

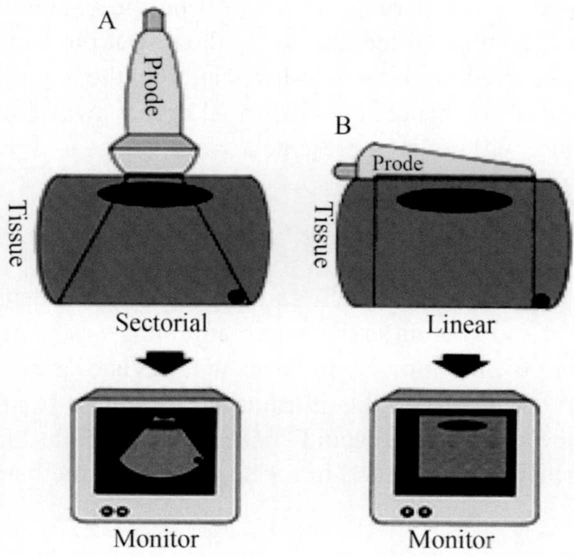

Sound Interaction with Tissue

The interaction of ultrasound with tissue causes a net energy loss called attenuation. When the ultrasound waves are transmitted into the body they will:

- Reflect
- Refract
- Absorb
- Scatter

All of these interactions together add up to attenuation.

Reflection

Diffuse reflectors: When a sound wave hits a relatively small interface, some of the wave will be transmitted through the interface and some will be reflected. When a reflector is small, we get what is termed diffuse reflection – the sound bounces around from reflector to reflector depending on the angle that the beam strikes, and eventually, partially returns to the transducer and is used to produce the image. These small reflectors assist in producing an appreciation of the texture of the organ being insonated.

Specular reflectors are large compared to the wavelength of the ultrasound beam. When they are insonated at 90° all of the reflected sound returns to the transducer, so they produce a very strong bright pixel on the image. Of course, some of the sound will be transmitted through to the rest of the tissue. If the specular reflector is insonated at an angle other than 90°, the angle of reflection will equal the angle of incidence; the beam will reflect away from the transducer, so that structure will not be represented on the image and will effectively disappear.

Refraction

It occurs when there is an impedance mismatch and the angle of incidence is not 90°. When the speed of sound is different in two adjoining tissues and the angle of incidence is not 90°, the ultrasound beam will deviate or bend, which can cause artifacts on the image. In this illustration, if the two tissues were the same impedance, the sound beam would continue in a straight line, but because there is a different speed of sound in the second tissue the beam deviates from its path.

Absorption

As the beam travels through tissue some of the energy contained within the beam is absorbed by the tissue as heat (bio effect). The overall effect on the ultrasound image is that the sound loses energy and the image quality is poorer as deeper tissues are tried for being penetrated. The higher the frequency the greater the absorption that occurs; this is a limiting factor for a transducer of a given frequency. All ultrasound transducers offer a compromise between high frequency high resolution and lower frequency but greater depth penetration into the tissue.

Scattering

It occurs when an ultrasound beam strikes an interface within the tissue. The pattern of the scattering depends on the size of the interface the beam strikes.

- If it strikes an interface much larger than the wavelength, we get reflection.
- If the interface is about the same size as the wavelength, the beam scatters randomly in all directions, depending on the orientation of the reflector to the beam and the phase of the wave which strikes the interface like diffuse reflections, we use this type of scattering to produce tissue information.
- If the interface is much smaller than the wavelength, we have Rayleigh scattering i.e., scattering of light by the particles present in the atmospherehencereflection is equal in all directions. It acts as a point

source of sound. RBCs scatter ultrasound in this manner; and this is utilized when obtaining a color or Doppler trace.

The echogenicity of a structure or an organ is not just determined by its density; it is determined by the number and type of reflectors within it, and the manner in which they interact with the sound waves.

Attenuation

Attenuation is not the same at absorption–attenuation is a combination of all the interactions of sound with tissue added together. The attenuation is equivalent to a loss of 1dB/cm / MHz (Gent p 74), but different tissues attenuate the ultrasound to varying degrees. In some tissue, such as muscleor nerves, the attenuation rate changes with the angle of insonation. These tissues are said to be anisotropic – the echogenicity of the structure will changewith the changing angle. One should always try to achieve an angle of 90° to the beam for all B-mode imaging.

Why we do ultrasonography of buck testes

Breeding soundness examination (BSE) of rams and bucks is performed by veterinarians as a service for producers to help identify males that may not be capable of settling females early in the breeding season and sire offspring with the genetic potential for rapid and efficient growth. In the routine BSE, palpation of the testis cannot assess with accuracy testicular parenchyma and presence of small lesions. Ultrasonography and testicular biometric parameters are a better approach for evaluation of the testes. In addition, testicular ultrasonography can be a important tool for the evaluation of scrotal circumference and testicular volume and prediction of fertility potential. To provide a basis for this BSE, this chapter presents a detailed overview of the anatomy of buck reproductive system and outlines the basis for ultrasonographic examination of the genital tract.

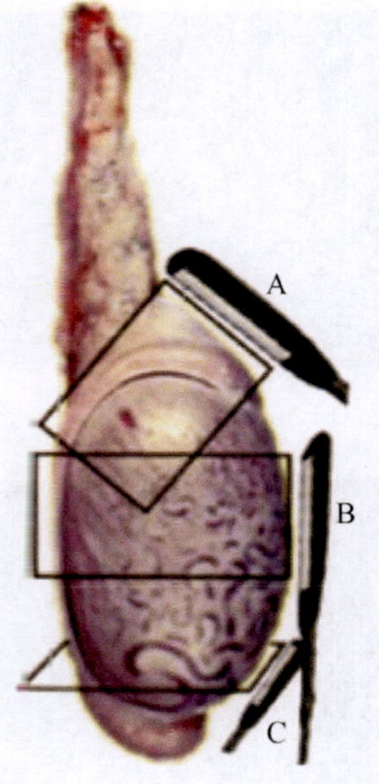

Fig 1: Ultrasonographic examination of the buck testicle with the use of linear probe for (A) Oblique, (B) Longitudinal (C) Transverse

USG of testes is done for the diagnosis of

1. Hydrocele
2. Orchitis

3. Peri-orchitis
4. Defects in spermatic cord
5. Testicular fibrosis
6. Abscess
7. Testicular calcification etc.

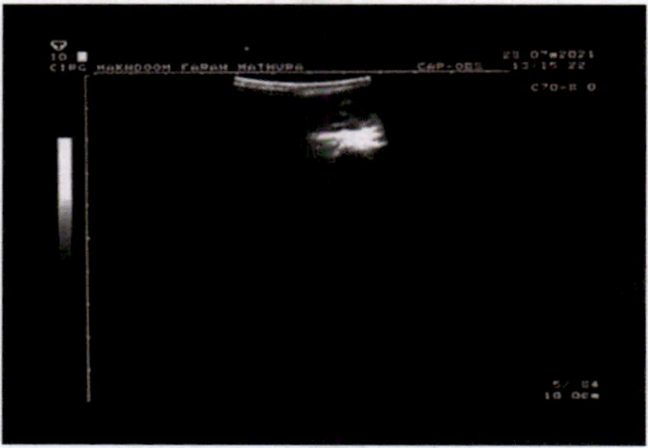
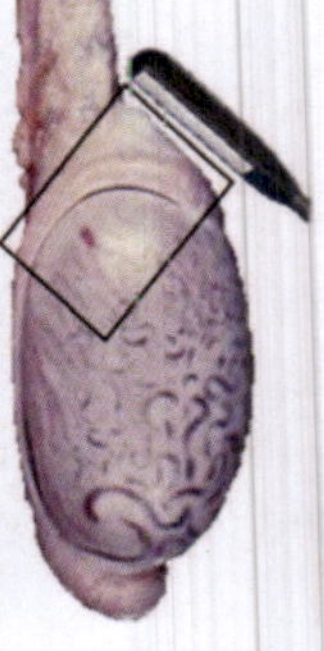
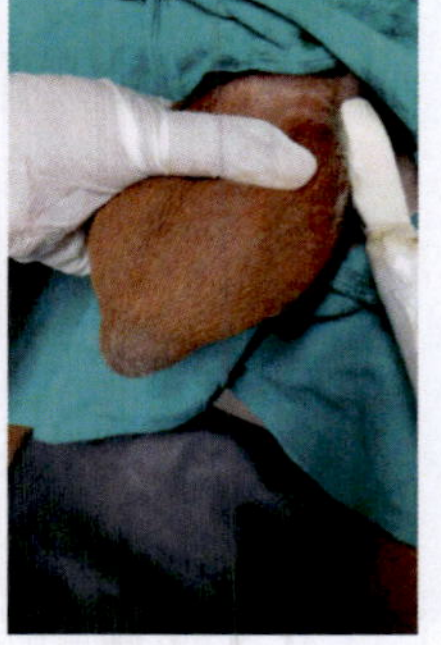

Fig. 2: Oblique sagittal scan of the testis at the level of the epididymis head to view the pampiniform plexus

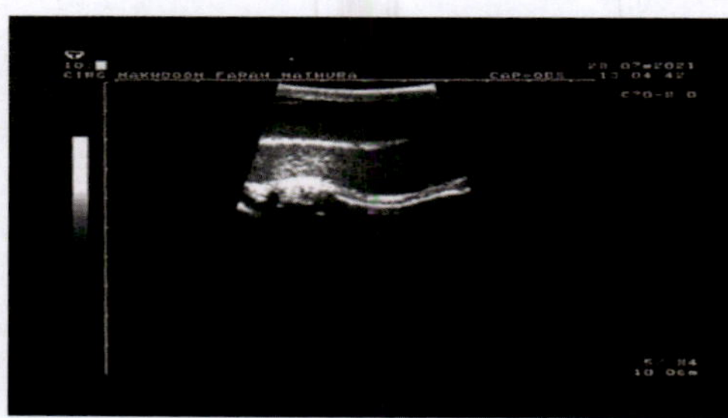
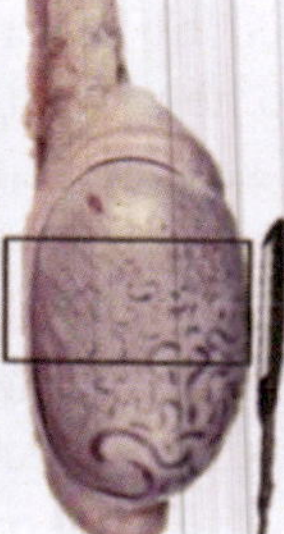
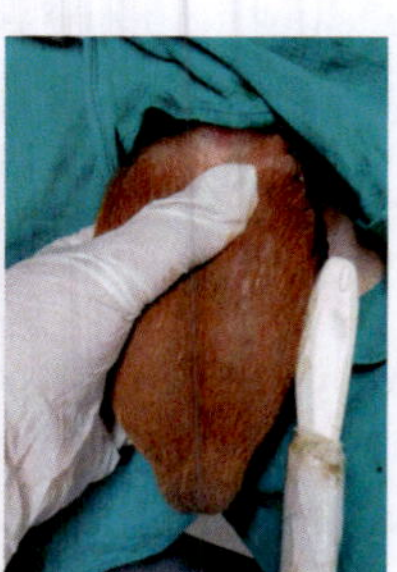

Fig. 3: Longitudinal scan of testes

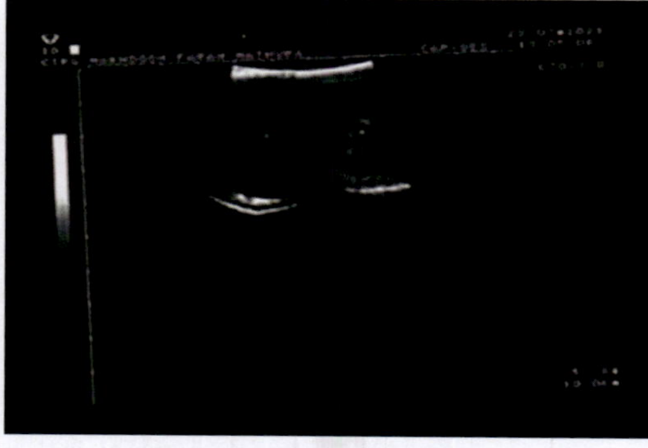
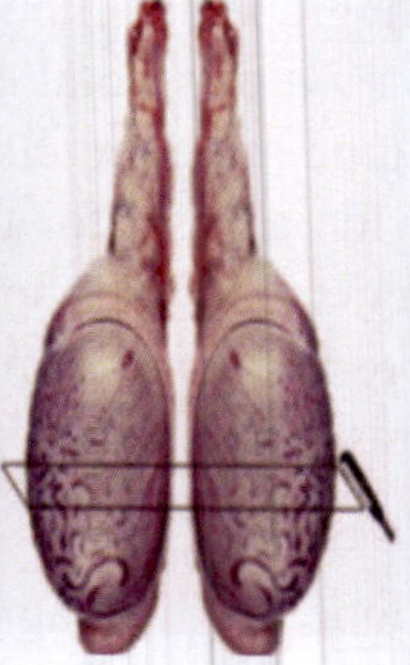
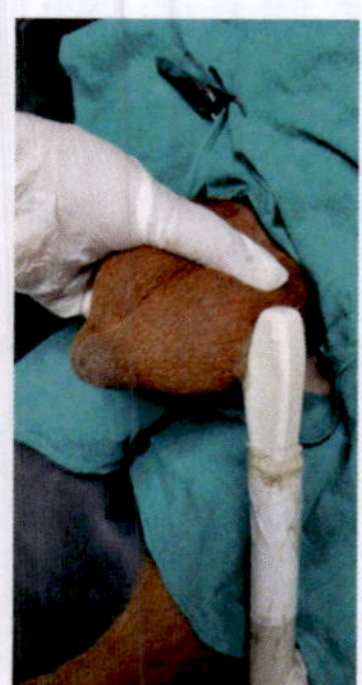

Fig. 4: Transverse scan of the testes

Ultrasonographic Artifacts

Artifacts result from a number of assumptions that the ultrasound machine has to make in order for it to produce an image. These assumptions include the following:

- Speed of sound is constant in soft tissue.
- All echoes detected by the transducer have come from the central axis of the beam.
- The ultrasound beam travels in straight lines.
- The time taken for a pulse to return to the transducer from a given interface is directly related to the distance from interface to reflector.
- An echo generated at an interface returns directly to the transducer without generating any secondary echoes.
- Rate of attenuation is constant. But these are assumptions and as a result, varying resultant appearances arepossible, such as:
- Echoes in a display that do not correspond with their position in the patient.
- Absence of echoes that should be displayed.
- Separate structures might display as a single joined structure.
- Brightness of echoes might not display correctly.
- A single structure can display as two separate structures.
- Thin membranes may display as being much thicker than in reality.

7

Shelter Management of Bucks in Different Production Systems

N. Ramachandran[1], B. Rai[2], Chetna Gangwar[2] and R. Pourouchottamane[2]

[1]Division of Bioenergetics and Environmental Sciences, ICAR- National Institute of Animal Nutrition and Physiology- 560030, Adugodi Bengaluru, Karnataka

[2]Animal Physiology and Reproduction Division, ICAR- Central Institute for Research on Goats, Makhdoom, Mathura, Uttar Pradesh

---

The goat rearing on extensive rearing system has been practiced since ancestry for livelihood and nutritional security of poor, landless and marginal farmers of our country with the flock size ranging from 2-10 goats. However, in the recent past, goat rearing is shifting towards semi-intensive and intensive rearing systems for commercial purposes with flock size ranging from 25 to 500. The goats reared in small flocks needs minimal housing facilities following the scientific principles with low-cost structures. On the other hand, elaborate housing is generally recommended for goats raised under large scale commercial production systems. Separate housing arrangements for different categories of animals viz. growers, pregnant females, lactating females, breeding males, etc. are to be ensured for rearing goats scientifically for harnessing maximum output sustainably.

The requirements of housing structures varies for different flock sizes and even may vary for one type of flock size under different rearing systems. Therefore, before deciding the type of housing facilities required, one must know few basic facts in housing requirements for different age categories of goats, irrespective of flock size, rearing systems, agro-climatic regions etc.

Table 1: Basic dimensions in minimum housing requirements

Description	Scientific requirement/recommendation
Orientation of shed	Sheds with long axis running east-west with generous provision for ventilation/air movement to help dry up the shed will be most suitable.
Length of shed	No restriction on the length of shed.
Breadth of shed	Normally between 6 m to 8m (Preferably not ≥ 20 feet).
Wall height	0.5-1.0m above ground on long side of shed & up to roof on width side of shed.
Roof height	2.7 m at eaves & 3.5 m at centre
Overhang of roof	0.75-1 m on both sides.
Gap between two sheds	6 m to 8m ((Preferably not < 20 feet).
Open paddocks	On one side of shed preferably south, if space constraints exits or on both sides.

Floor space

Age / Category of goats	Covered area (m^2/goat)	Open paddock (m^2/goat)
0 - 3-month-old male kids	0.2-0.25	0. 4-0.5
3 - 6-month-old male kids	0.5-0.75	1.0-1.5
6 - 12-month-old male kids	0.75-1.0	1.5-2.0
Yearling male goats (above 12 months)	1.00	2.00
Adult Bucks	1.5-2.0	3.0-4.0

Ventilation space

Season	Ventilation space
Hot dry	70% of floor area
Hot humid	Longer sides be kept totally open
Cool	2-10% of floor area (or provide flexible ventilation. i.e., Maximum between 10 am to 4 pm, and closing the ventilation space between 4 pm to 10 am.
Comfortable	25% of floor area

Floor type: Clay/soil floor in regions with predominant hot-dry climate and slatted floors for hot–humid weather conditions.

Roof type: Thatch roof, corrugated cemented sheets or galvanized iron sheets and any other alternate roofing materials, usage depends on fund available and weather conditions.

Shelter Surroundings: Maintain the green vegetation and greenery all-round the shed (grass, hedges, shrubs, shrubs, tree) adjacent to the goat shelters.

Hedges and shrubs planted at a distance of 2 m from the building and their height should be below the height of opening for ventilation but toward west side height. Creepers over the roof shall be tried.

Bedding: Locally available 2-4 inches thick soft dry grasses unsuitable for feeding (straw, hay, dried corn stalks, corn cobs, peanut hulls, cottonseed hulls, oat hulls, sawdust, wood shavings, wood chips, pine shavings, sand, paper products, peat, hemp and leaves) shall be used especially for 0-3 months old kids and milking does.

Shelter requirements for bucks

In general, the goats reared under **extensive free range rearing systems**, the male kids and adult bucks are raised in same flock and no separate housing is provided for male goats even the flock strength up to 200. However, in semi-intensive and intensively reared flocks, male kids are separated from female kids at 3 months age and are reared in separate enclosures lifelong. If the farm having 10 goats, the male required for breeding is one adult male; for 25 goats, one adult male and one young male of lesser age; for 50 goats, two adult males and one young male of lesser age; for 100 goats, three adult males and two young males of lesser age is generally recommended. As per the floor space requirement, farm with 10 goats need minimum 9m x 3m shed with single slope roof is required. Out of which 18 m^2 may be allowed for does, 4 m^2 for buck, 4 m^2 for kids having separate temporary partitions inside the shed. If the flock size is up to 25 goats, minimum 12m x 6m shed with either single or double slope roof in covered area and double the space area for open paddocks is required. Out of which 36 m^2 may be allowed for adult does follow by 24 m^2 for growing kids inclusive of temporary partitions for kids up to 3 months and on other end of shed, 12m^2 for bucks. The provisions (gate) for crossing each partition in covered and open area should also be required for efficient time saving and space utilization.

The importance of goat shelter starts from medium goat farms, where without shelter, the optimum economic return cannot be achieved. If the flock size is up to 50 goats, a minimum 25m x 6m shed with double slope roof in covered area and double the space area for open paddocks is required for medium sized goat flocks. Out of which 45 m^2 may be allowed for adult does follow by 30 m^2 for adult lactating does, 12 m^2 for kids up to 3 months, 18 m^2 for male growing kids, 18 m^2 for female growing and on other end of shed, 15m^2 for bucks. The additional 12 m^2 adjacent to buck pen without open area may be provided for store. The provisions (gate) for crossing each partition in covered and open area should also be required for efficient time saving and space utilization.

The goat farming is gradually taking a shape of industry from farming practices especially by educated and unemployed youths, retired and IT professionals. Therefore, for large scale farming, permanent shelter is essentially required for taking up the goat rearing in the form of commercial enterprise. A minimum of two sheds facing each other is required for 100 goats with followers. One shed with 25m x 6m shed with double slope roof in covered area and double the space area for open paddocks is required for does and suckling kids. Out of which 30 m^2 may be allowed for adult does follow by 54 m^2 for adult pregnant does, 54 m^2 for adult lactating does, 12 m^2 for kids up to 3 months on other end of the shed adjacent to lactating does pen. The second shed with same dimension as that of first shed is required for bucks, growing male kids, growing female kids, store, office etc. Out of which 30 m^2 may be allowed for 18 m^2 for adult bucks, 45 m^2 male growing kids, 45 m^2 for female growing kids with the double space in open paddock is required. On other end of second shed, 24 m^2 room for store and 18 m^2 for shed office may be planned without open paddocks. The provisions (gate) for crossing each partition in covered and open area should also be required for efficient time saving and space utilization. Additionally, 18 m^2 sick animal pen and 18 m^2 clinic near office for critical care, 40 m^2 quarantine shed in covered area having double open space at least 100 meters away from main shed, 250 m^2 bhusa godown having double slope with 7 m height at centre and 5.5 m height at eave is essentially required for easy unloading from truck. In medium and larger flocks, farm gate, farm roads, fencing, dipping tank, foot bath etc. are also needed for taking up routine and periodic activities timely. If the flock size is more than 100 with followers, the same facilities need to be expanded like number of sheds, size of pens etc on case-to-case basis. The buck pen should be adjacent to dry females pen to induce estrus cycle; however, it should be away from pregnant animal's pen.

In medium sized goat farms under extensive rearing system, kids are housed in temporary enclosure in small groups and maintained in shed itself till 3 months age and thereafter, kids are allowed for grazing along with does for shorter duration nearest to the shed i.e. during day time, kids enclosure/paddock shall be made in the surrounding of goat shelter where small agro-forestry (trees and grasses grown) for grazing is developed and feeding arrangements should be under the trees and after 4-5 months age, kids shall be allowed for grazing in group of 40-50 kids initially for 2-3 hours in nearby the goat shed. The full time grazing of kids along with does is suggested for kids above 6 months age. If goats are reared under semi-intensive and intensive rearing system, kids are housed along with their does in individual cages of minimum 1.5' x 1.5' size for first week of their life and thereafter, they are housed in temporary enclosure inside the permanent shelter in a group of 40-50 kids of similar age and body size. After weaning, male and female kids are housed separately till 12 months of age. The floor of the kids house should be clean and dry as far as possible. During winter, 4-inches thick bedding is to be used to avoid soil licking in suckling kids. The bedding materials have to be removed daily, dry in sun light and reuse in the kid's enclosure daily till the foul smell starts. If it fouls, replace with new bedding materials. Use lime dusting in soil floor to remove excess moisture and destroy disease causing agents. The place of kid's enclosure should be rotated with the permanent shelter at monthly intervals to reduce coccidial load. Alternatively, where the floor is not possible to get dry or worm (coccidial) load used to be high, slatted wooden/bamboo/plastic floor materials shall be easily used as bedding at 6-inch height from floor. The long side of the shelter should be protected with gunny bags and 4 thick thatch panels made from locally available materials to keep the kids warm during peak winter nights. The adult male and female goats (above 1 year age) are housed in group separately. Adult female goats are housed in groups as per physiological stages like dry, pregnant and lactating goats for giving special care and feeding arrangements which shall be either fixed along the walls or separate recommended movable feeders shall be used to reduce wastage in the shed. The concentrate store, bhusa store, sick animal pen and quarantine pen, office etc should also available on large sized flock. During grazing hours, male and female flocks should be grazed separately and special care should be given to avoid stray mating. The temporary shelter, paddocks and watering tanks in grazing field shall be tried to have split grazing (rest during peak sun light hours) and to avoid energy loss due to excess walking.

Individual buck pens for higher semen production

The performance of a goat flock largely depends upon the kind of buck used for breeding rather than individual doe as one buck is used to serve several hundred does. Hence, selection of a superior breeding buck and optimum management of individual buck is critical in harvesting good quality semen with optimum freezability. It has been observed that managing breeding males of different ages, breed, body size in groups increase abnormal behaviours/ vices that leads to loss of superior germplasm (Ramachandran et al., 2006, 2007, 2012). Therefore, it was recommended as one of the control measures for vices that the bucks should be housed individually rather than rearing them in group for feeding and management. Ramachandran et al. (2020) prepared a design and layout plan of individual housing of bucks in any frozen semen station for minimum 30 adult breeding bucks, 6 bucks in each breed covering 4-5 breeds in any particular agro-climatic zone. Bucks after screening for breeding soundness evaluation and semen freezability, the selected bucks are maintained in individual buck shed. The bucks are maintained under stall feeding conditions under individual feeding system. If they are maintained under semi-intensive rearing system, bucks should be stall-fed individually during peak breeding season for natural mating and /or suitable peak semen collection periods. The total space requirement for constructing shed for individual housing of 30 adult breeding bucks is calculated as 300 sq. meter. As per the proposed two-sided face to face shed design with the required total floor space for 30 bucks, the doubled sided shed dimension shall be 15m x8 m (3m + 2m + 3m) in covered area with 15m x 6m open paddocks on both the side. The minimum wall height at width side in covered area in a double-sided roof should be of 3.5 m at centre and 2.7 m at eave and the walls should be up to roof in width side. The wall height at length side of shed in covered area should be 1.0-1.5 m from the floor. The height of partition walls between individual buck enclosure should be minimum 1.5 m from floor and should not facilitate visibility among bucks to avoid sexual stimulation and to induce aggressiveness and libido during semen collection/mating. However, the partition walls should not hinder the free air movement so as to keep the floor dry and in hygienic conditions. The floor shall be of soil type, however, to avoid dust particles and other contaminations in semen samples, the soil floor shall be covered with wooden slats at 6-12 inches height from the floor. The covered area of 8 m width in double sloped shed shall be protected with roofing sheets having length of 2.44m (8ft) in two rows on each side for having minimum 1m overhang of roof on both side of covered area is possible to avoid rain water entry and dampness of floor. The ridge ventilation in double sloped double sided shed is recommended to avoid thermal and humid stress to bucks. The entry for each individual buck enclosure in the form of gate is designed in covered area in such a way that they are opened and closed in central passage. However, this can be modified by designing gate for entry via each open paddock in outer boundary on both sides.

8

Feeding Management of Bucks for Improving Reproductive Efficiency

Ravindra Kumar, Mohd. Arif, D.L. Gupta and C. Gangwar

Division of ANM&PT, ICAR-Central Institute for Research on Goats Makhdoom, Farah - 281 122, Uttar Pradesh

Nutrition is the key factor affecting the production as well as the reproduction efficiency in all the animals therefore proper and balanced nutrition is the prerequisite to attain and utilize the full reproductive potential of the animals. All the nutrients like energy, protein, minerals and vitamins need to be properly balanced in the diet of animals. Energy and protein are the major nutrients required in the greatest amounts and should be in the topmost priority in order to optimize reproduction. Although minerals and vitamins are required in low amount, but very much essential as a cofactor and coenzymes in the reproductive process of the animals and deficiency of these nutrients might affect the overall reproductive efficiency of the animals.

Nutritional factors affecting reproduction

Energy: Insufficient energy intake is probably the single most important nutritional factor related to poor reproductive function in animals. Metabolic priorities for energy are in following order 1) basal metabolism, 2) activity, 3) growth, 4) energy reserves, 5) pregnancy, 6) lactation, 7) additional energy reserves, 8) estrous cycles and initiation of pregnancy, and 9) excess energy reserves. In case of low energy intake, reproductive function is compromised because available energy is directed towards meeting minimum energy reserves and milk production. Restricting energy intake during late gestation increases the length of postpartum anestrous and reduces subsequent pregnancy rate.

However, excessive energy intake during late lactation and the dry period can cause problems which lower reproductive efficiency in the next lactation. When animals are fed inadequate amounts of energy, they reach sexual maturity later. If energy deficient rations are fed that have begun to have normal estrous cycles, they may stop cycling. An excessive energy intake during the late lactation and dry periods can lead to "fat cow" problems. Cows that are over-conditioned when they calve have a higher incidence of retained placenta, more uterine infections and more cystic ovaries. They also have a higher incidence of metabolic disorders and have a greater tendency to go off feed. All of these problems can result in poor reproductive performance.

Protein: The effect of dietary protein on reproduction is complex. Prolonged inadequate protein intake has been reported to reduce reproductive performance. Reproductive performance may be impaired if protein is fed in amounts that greatly exceed the requirements. Over-feeding of DIP either as protein or urea has been associated with decreased pregnancy rates in female. It appears that exposure to high levels of ammonia or urea may impair maturation of oocytes and subsequent fertilization or maturation of developing embryos. However, supplying adequate energy for excretion of excess ammonia or urea may prevent decreases in fertility. However, regardless of a possible effect on reproductive performance, overfeeding protein should be discouraged simply on an economic basis. It is costly and wasteful. Urea is added to some dairy rations as a source of nitrogen which the rumen bacteria can convert into protein.

Minerals: Minerals are important for all physiological processes in animals including reproduction. Mineral deficiencies and imbalances are often cited as causes of poor reproduction. It is clear that adequate amounts of minerals must be provided, but little is known about the effects of marginal deficiencies and imbalances. The same is true of excessive intakes of minerals which may indeed be harmful. Minerals are required in smaller quantities but they play very crucial role. They are part of structural components of tissues, act as electrolytes in fluids, and play critical roles in the proper functioning of enzymes or hormones. Trace elements are required for all physiological functions, and support optimal growth, health condition, the immune system, productivity and reproduction. An inadequate supply of trace elements will lead to a deficiency and cause biochemical dysfunction, disturbed physiological functions or structural disorders. Generally, it is observed that single trace element deficiency is rare while deficiency of combined element is more common. Some trace elements are particularly important for ruminants, for example for rumen digestion (Co, Cu, Mo), performance (Co, Cu, Fe, I, Mn, Mo, Se, Zn), fertility (Co, Cu, I, Mn, Se and Zn). The trace elements which are very much essential from reproduction point of view, their major function along with deficiency symptoms are presented in table 1.

Table 1: Minerals their function and deficiency symptoms related to reproduction

Element	Proposed mechanism/ function	Deficiency symptoms
Zinc	Component of various enzymes	Decrease oocyte maturation, Anovulation and spermatogenesis
Selenium	Decrease ROS/oxidative stress	Retained placenta, still birth
Iron	Cell growth/function,LH & FSH secretion	Infertility, Anovulation
Copper	Component of cuprous enzymes	Decrease Libido
Cobalt	Component of B_{12}	Delay in onset of puberty, decreased conception rate
Manganese	Cholesterol synthesis	testicular atrophy in males and impaired ovulation in females
Molybdenum	Oxidase enzyme system	Decreased libido and conception rate
Bromine	Collagen formation, halogen replacement	Decrease tissue integrity
Chromium	Helps in gametogenesis	Early embryonic death

Keeping the importance of minerals in the physiological and reproductive processes of animals it is always recommended to add mineral mixture at the rate of 2% in the concentrate mixture for the animals.

Vitamins: The vitamin requirements of ruminants are met by a combination of rumen and tissue synthesis, natural feeds and feed supplementations. Most commercial concentrates contain supplemental vitamins so the probability of infertility due to a vitamin deficiency is greatly reduced. When commercial concentrates are not fed, vitamin supplements should be provided. All B-complex vitamins are synthesized in the rumen under normal circumstances. Fat soluble vitamins such as Vitamin A, Vitamin D and vitamin E are dietary essential in case of ruminants. When feed intake is restricted and (or) low quality forage is fed to control or reduce body condition. To ensure adequate intake, vitamins and minerals should be fed in small amounts of low energy concentrates or mixed in a complete dry cow ration.

Feed formulation for growing and adult buck

Growing bucks: Depending upon the land and pasture available, bucks can be reared on grazing with supplementation or stall-fed system. This will reduce the cost of production and farmers can get more benefit. Normally growing goats/ bucks of 4-12 months of age consume dry matter equal to 4% of their body weight. The ration of goats/bucks should provide 12-14% of crude protein and 60-65% total digestible nutrients. When good pasture is available, they can be allowed for grazing for 7-8 hours. In this case supplementation of 100-200gram concentrate mixture having 1-2% mineral mixture provides good growth and economic benefit to farmers. If grazing is not available then concentrate mixture along with leguminous straw and green fodder is good option to rear growing goats for more economic returns. The concentrate mixture can be formulated by mixing maize (57%), ground nut cake (20%), wheat bran (20%), mineral mixture (2%) and salt (1%).

Adult bucks: Depending upon the nutrient availability in the pasture and time of grazing, the amount of green fodder and concentrate mixture can be modified. The concentrate mixture can be prepared by mixing grains like maize, barley, bajra (55-60%), De-oiled cake like ground nut cake, linseed cake etc (15-20%), wheat bran (15-20%), mineral mixture (2%) and salt (1%). When good pasture is available, they can be allowed for grazing for 5-6 hours, in addition to this supplementation of 300-400 gm straw, 1000-1500gm green fodder and 500 gm concentrate mixture (during breeding season) provides good growth and economic benefit to farmers.

Effect of Azolla feeding on bucks

Azolla a free-floating aquatic fern which fixes atmospheric nitrogen in association with nitrogen fixing blue green algae *Anabaena azollae*, making it an excellent source of protein for livestock. This can be used as a part of feed or as a supplemental source of protein and minerals in the ration of bucks. Azolla in the complete feed can reduce the cost of feed of goat there by increasing the profits from goat rearing to the farmers. Azolla was found to contain 78-80% organic matter, 17-22% crude protein, 2-3% crude fat and 12-15% crude fibre on dry matter basis. The NDF and ADF of azolla recorded were 45-47% and 30- 33%, respectively. Sodium, potassium, calcium was 0.60%, 0.73%, 0.11% while Copper and zinc was 16.12ppm and 71.47ppm respectively indicating azolla as a good source of macro as well as micro minerals. Fresh azolla can be fed to growing and adult bucks. Fresh azolla harvested can be mixed with straw and fed to the bucks. The rate of incorporation of azolla should be 50-100 gm/day in growing animals and 100-200 gm/day in the adult animals. Experiment was conducted on feeding of fresh azolla in bucks found that azolla supplementation improved reaction time and progressive motility in Barbari bucks. There is also positive effect of azolla supplementation on semen freezability. There was significant improvement in post thaw motility, live sperm count, acrosomal integrity and hypo-osmotic swelling positive spermatozoa on dietary azolla supplementation to breeding bucks. So azolla feeding improved the quality and freezability of semen favouring the use in artificial insemination program.

Conclusion

Nutrition has a profound effect on reproductive potential in all living species. Energy and protein are the nutrients required in the greatest amounts and should be first priority in developing nutritional programs to optimize reproduction. Minerals and vitamins must be balanced in the diet to optimize reproductive performance. Azolla contain good amount of protein, fibre, all essential macro and micro minerals and lesser amounts of ADF and NDF. Feeding of fresh azolla to bucks improved reaction time and progressive motility and have also positive effect on semen freezability.

9

Health Management of Breeding Bucks

Ashok Kumar[1], Chetna Gangwar[2] and Vinay Chaturvedi[1]

[1]Division of Animal Health, ICAR-Central Institute for Research on Goats Makhdoom, Farah-281 122, Mathura, Uttar Pradesh, India
[2]Department of Animal Reproduction, ICAR-Central Institute for Research on Goats Makhdoom, Farah-281 122, Mathura, Uttar Pradesh, India

Occasionally some diseases can be noticed in male animals, which are responsible for the reduced reproductive performance of the bucks. Sometimes these diseases can damage or obstruct the male reproductive passage and responsible for the infertility and sterility in the bucks. This type of infertility may be associated with pathology of testes, epididymis, vas deferens, accessory sex glands, and urethra or may be associated with abnormal semen production due to congenital or hereditary causes or due to acquired causes.

Cryptorchidism

Normally the testes are situated in the scrotum at or soon after birth through descent of testes. Failure of one or both the testes to descend into scrotum at appropriate time is known as cryptorchidism. Unilateral cryptorchidism is more common and the affected males are near normally fertile because of normal production of semen from the testis located in the scrotum. Cryptorchidism, if bilateral, results in sterility. In retained or cryptorchic testes, spermatogenesis is inhibited because of elevated temperature of the affected testis cryptorchid testis is usually small in size, soft and flaccid. The cryptorchidism is seen in all domestic species. It is most commonly seen in stallions, boars and dog, less commonly seen in rams and bucks. The cryptorchidism is a hereditary condition and such animal should not be used for breeding.

Imperfect Descent of Testis

Sometimes in animals, the testes though not cryptorchid are located fairly high in the scrotum and are somewhat horizontal. Such animals are called "high flankers". This may due to attachment of cremaster muscle to the caudal aspect of testis, fixation of the lower end of scrotum to the perineal region or lower attachment of gubernaculum. In such animals, because of imperfect thermos regulatory mechanisms, the testes show degeneration and atrophy and the fertility is impaired. The condition might be genetic in nature.

Scrotal or Inguinal Hernia

Scrotal or inguinal hernias are reported commonly in stallions and boars. A large scrotal hernia would greatly interfere with the testicular function of the affected side because of elevated temperature and increased pressure on the testes caused by herniated loop of the intestine. In smaller degree of inguinal hernia, there are greater chances of strangulation of the intestine. If mating is allowed by the male, there are fair chances that due to increased abdominal pressure during the coitus, the loop of the intestine may be forced through inguinal opening and thus the condition may worsen. The condition is considered to be of hereditary in origin. Animal with inguinal hernia be castrated and should not be used for breeding.

Testicular Hypoplasia

The testicular hypoplasia is a unilateral or bilateral condition noted at the time of puberty or later. The condition is commonly noted in bulls, rams, bucks, boars and stallions. Testicular hypoplasia is a congenital and hereditary condition caused by single recessive autosomal gene with incomplete penetration. The condition is due to lack of or marked reduction in spermatogonia in the gonad during the fetal life. There may be (1) failure of germ cells to develop in the yolk sac, (2) failure of germ cells to migrate to the gonad, (3) failure of the germ cells to multiply in the gonad and (4) extensive degeneration of the germ cells after they have reached the gonads.

Lowered conception rates are associated with bilateral testicular hypoplasia. Only in bilateral complete testicular hypoplasia, the animals are sterile. In most of the cases of testicular hypoplasia, the sexual desire is excellent and the coitus is prompt. The affected testes are reduced in size and are usually firmer. The affected bucks have small and firm epididymis indicating reduction in spermatogenesis as well as in gonadal sperm reserves. The semen picture is characterized by low concentration of spermatozoa, low motility, high incidence of proximal protoplasmic droplets and abnormal spermatozoa. In bilateral cases the semen is usually clear and watery with only few or no spermatozoa. Giant cells (or multinucleated cells with 6-8 nuclei) and medusa cells (or ciliated cells) from different tubules may be observed in the ejaculate. These multinucleated cells are the result of incomplete maturation division of the primary spermatocytes. The nuclei divide but the cytoplasmic divisions are not complete. The development of the other genital organs (except testes) is normal. Histologically, the seminiferous tubules are very much underdeveloped with only the basal layer of the cells being present. Varying degree of spermatogenesis may be present from spermatogonia, spermatocytes and spermatids to abnormal and normal spermatozoa.

The prognosis in testicular hypoplasia is poor since the condition is hereditary. The affected animals should not be used for breeding purpose.

The treatment of testicular hypoplasia is not successful and the animals should be culled.

Testicular Degeneration

It is estimated that 75 to 80% of the testicular pathology is related to testicular degeneration. The epithelium of the testis is most sensitive to any adverse influence. Generalized disease process brings about bilateral testicular degeneration and the local testicular lesions bring about unilateral testicular degeneration. The testicular degeneration is very rapid (may be within hours or days) but the testicular regeneration process is very slow and it may take several weeks to several months for recovery. Further when the basal layer of the germinal epithelium (including spermatogonia and Sertoli cells) is destroyed, regeneration is not possible and the animal becomes sterile. The changes in testicular degeneration are almost common in all species e.g., reduced concentration of spermatozoa, reduced motility of spermatozoa, increased number of abnormal spermatozoa, atrophic seminiferous tubules and testes smaller and softer. Such changes would depend upon the degree of degeneration. In chronic cases of testicular degeneration, the testis may become firm due to fibrosis and even there may be deposition of calcium in areas peripheral to the rate testis.

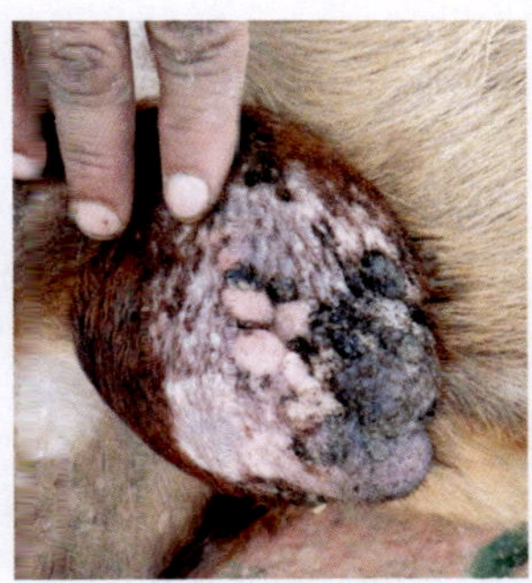

Testicular Degeneration

The various causes for testicular degeneration are

1. **Thermal influence:** Prolonged elevated body temperature as in certain infectious disease, prolonged high environmental temperature particularly associated with high humidity, direct heating of scrotum, increase in the scrotal temperature due to any other cause e.g., irritants, dermatitis, cryptorchidism and ectopic testes cause testicular degeneration. Summer infertility in exotic bulls and rams is a common phenomenon.

2. **Vascular lesion of the testes**: Interference in the blood circulation of the testes e.g., torsion of testes, presence of strongly larvae in the testicular artery in the horse, varicoceles of the spermatic vein may cause infraction and may affect heat regulatory mechanism leading to degenerative changes in the testis.
3. **Irradiation**: Irradiation produces interference with spermatogenesis and spermatogonia, spermatids and spermatocytes are injured. The most sensitive are spermatocytes, while the Leydig cells and Sertoli cells are quiet resistant to radiation. The first change is the increase in the number of abnormal spermatozoa and then there is decrease in the concentration of the spermatozoa.
4. **Hormonal cause**: Tumors of the anterior pituitary gland or hypothalamus interfere with the production of gonadotropic hormones. This is seen most commonly in dog and rarely in other animals. In dog these tumors are also associated with testicular atrophy and degeneration and with obesity and are referred to as "dystrophia adiposogenitalis". Sertoli cell tumors produce excessive amount of estrogen. Leydig cells tumors produce excessive amount of testosterone and estrogen. These excessive steroids may suppress the production of FSH and may cause testicular degeneration.
5. **Age effects:** Old age has been reported to be associated with rather permanent and progressive testicular degeneration nearly in all species of animals e.g. dogs over 10 years of age, cats over 12 years of age and bulls over 8-10 years of age. This phenomenon is affected by disease, genetic and managemental factors.
6. **Trauma, stress or disease:** Trauma, stress or disease factors may cause rapid testicular degeneration in males e.g., long duration shipping under stress of heat or cold, severe fatigue, traumatic gastritis, internal abscesses, severe and multiple contusions, severe arthritis, severe myiasis (disease of tissue or cavity by larvae and flies), laminitis, foot rot, traumatic lesions of testis and scrotum.
7. **Localized or systemic infectious diseases:** Localized or systemic infectious diseases are common causes of testicular degeneration. Infections causing orchitis or epididymitis as a normal inflammatory process produce heat, oedema and congestion etc. The thick and firm tunica albuginea restrict normal swelling of the testis and testicular degeneration occurs. Any disease localized in the testis may cause abscessation and testicular degeneration. *Brucella abortus,*

Mycobacterium tuberculosis, Corynebacterium pyogenes, Actinomyces etc. produce orchitis, epididymitis, testicular degeneration and testicular fibrosis. Severe obstructive lesions affecting the efferent ducts may cause back pressure resulting in testicular degeneration. Sporadic infections e.g., *Streptococci*, *Staphylococci, E. coli*, *Proteus and Pseudomonas*, all may cause orchitis in animals.

8. **Diseases causing fever, debilitation, inanition and loss of body weight:** Diseases causing fever, debilitation, inanition and loss of body weight etc. may cause testicular degeneration (e.g., pneumonia, severe paresis)

9. **Nutrition:** Underfeeding and malnutrition producing debility and loss of body weight may suppress the release of gonadotropic hormones from the anterior pituitary gland and may cause testicular degeneration. Severe Vit. A deficiency may produce testicular degeneration. High feeding levels and obesity generally do not affect the semen quality in normal males but it does affect willingness to mount.

10. **Poisons:** Various poisons may adversely affect the germinal epithelium. Dipping of bucks in arsenic solution causes degeneration of seminiferous tubules. Antimony compounds (for treating heart worms) in dog causes temporary infertility. Chlorinated naphthalene produces testicular degeneration in bulls and rams. Alkylating agents, Cadmium chloride and Amphotericin B produce testicular degeneration with Freund's adjuvant has been reported to cause testicular degeneration.

11. **Autoimmunization:** Experimentally (not in natural causes) autoimmunization with s/c injections of autologous testicular material together with Freund's adjuvant has been reported to cause testicular degeneration.

12. **Testicular tumors:** The testicular tumors may originate from interstitial cells. Sertoli cells and from germinal epithelium. Usually, the tumors are observed in old age. The large tumors may cause testicular degeneration either due to their compressing effect or due to excess of steroids produced by interstitial or Sertoli cell tumors.

The signs of testicular degeneration are almost similar in all species and may range from mild to severe depending upon the cause, duration and the degree of degeneration. The testicular size is usually reduced because of the atrophy of seminiferous tubules. In acute orchitis, inflammatory conditions, obstruction of the efferent tubules and testicular degeneration, the testicular size is usually increased.

The consistency of the testes is generally soft and yielding in testicular degeneration. Nearly 80% of the testes is composed of seminiferous tubules and their contents. In mild cases, consistency differs only slightly. In acute cases there is tense swelling and enlarged with pain and heat. The chronic cases may show fibrosis and calcification.

The sex drive is usually not affected except in painful conditions of in severely debilitating conditions (Leydig cells are more resistant to stress factors than the cells of germinal epithelium).

The semen picture is helpful in diagnosis of testicular conditions or in severely debilitating that a wide period (60-70 days in bull, 40-45 days in stallion, 60-70 days in ram, 50-60 days in boar and 60-70 days in Dog) is required for spermatogenesis until sperms are ejaculated. Hence it is necessary to take several samples at weekly or greater intervals for diagnosing testicular degeneration. Moreover, semen samples taken after a long period of sexual rest may be misleading as such samples, are of poor quality and have increased number of dead spermatozoa. The semen may be watery and translucent with azoospermia (no sperms) and oligozoospermia (reduced sperm concentration). The sperm motility is reduced because of increased percentage of abnormal cells, dead cells and poorly viable cells. There is an increase in abnormal heads, middle pieces and tails. The occurrence of large number of primary abnormalities are more indicative of testicular degeneration (e.g. macrocephalic sperm, microcephalic sperm, short broad heads, elongated narrow heads, pear shaped heads, double heads, double middle pieces and tails, swelling of middle pieces, Kinked or coiled middle pieces and tails and abasically attached middle pieces). Giant or multi nucleated cells are increased in testicular degeneration. The fertility may vary from only slight reduction in conception rate to severe infertility.

Nomenclature in semen analysis

Parameter	Criterion	Nomenclature
Volume	No volume Reduced volume increased volume	Aspermia Hypospermia Hyperspermia
Sperm concentration	Zero concentration Normal concentration Reduced concentration Increased concentration	Azoospermia Normozoospermia Oligozoospermia Polyzoospermia
Sperm motility Sperm viability Abnormal sperms	Decreased motilityAll dead sperms High percentage of abnormal sperm	Asthenozoospermia Necrozoospermia Teratozoospermia

The prognosis in testicular degeneration is variable depending upon the causative factors, duration and the degree of degeneration and the age of the animal. In young animals, in slight and mild cases and with transient and correctable causes, the prognosis is fair to good. The prognosis is poor in chronic cases, advanced testicular degeneration, severe orchitis, abscessation, and biliterate tumors and in cases with severe secondary lesions in the epididymis, accessory glands and vas deferens. Severe testicular degeneration leads to fibrosis and calcification and recovery is never possible.

The treatment of testicular degeneration consists of correction of the causative factors/alleviation of causative factor and sexual rest Some mild cases can be treated. Some cases may require a balanced diet supplemented with Vit. A and quality proteins. In cases of acute orchitis, sexual rest and broad range antibiotics together with glucocorticoids may be given. Testosterone, FSH preparations and Thyroxin have not been found to be of therapeutic value in the cases of testicular degeneration and hypoplasia. Further, gonadotropic hormones need to be given for months and these should be derived from the same biological source to prevent developing of antihormones. If the orchitis is unilateral, affected testis may be removed to hasten recovery and to save breeding life of valuable animals. Brucella infected bulls or boars should not be used in Brucella free animals either naturally or artificially. Testes with tumors should be removed to prevent secondary tumors due to metastases. Testicular tumors are common in cryptorchid testes and cryptorchid testes should be removed in the young age.

Orchitis

Orchitis denotes inflammation of the testes. It is caused mostly by bacterial infections (e.g., Brucella abortus) and by some viral agents (e.g. Epivag in African countries). It is generally haematogenous in origin. It may be caused from wounds penetrating the scrotal sac and several infectious agents may be involved in causing orchitis e.g., *Streptococci, Staphylococci, C. pyogenes., proteus, E. coli, P. aeruginosa* etc. It may also be caused by descending infections from accessory sex glands through vas deferens.

In acute cases, the scrotum becomes hot, painful and oedematous. There may be rise in body temperature and anorexia.

The treatment would consist of sexual rest, antiseptic dressing, application of ice packs and broad range antibiotics with glucocorticoids by parenteral routes. Brucella infected bucks should never be used on brucella- free- flock either naturally or through artificial insemination.

Testicular Fibrosis

Testicular fibrosis is usually the end result of testicular inflammation and testicular degeneration. In testicular fibrosis, the Leydig cells and seminiferous tubules are replaced by fibrous tissue. Some areas of necrosis, calcification and lymphocytic infiltration may also be seen. The ejaculates are watery and contain few or no sperms.

Testicular Calcification

Testicular calcification is associated with testicular degeneration and is usually bilateral. In one study 9.55% incidence of testicular calcification was recorded in male buffalo collected from abattoir. Such testes are hard.

Testicular Neoplasms

This does not appear to be common in bucks. Testicular tumors are common in dogs. The testicular tumors originate from interstitial cells, Sertoli cells and germinal epithelium. Usually, the testicular tumors are observed in old age. The large testicular tumors cause degeneration either due to their compressing effect or due to excess of steroid hormones produced by interstitial cell/Sertoli cell tumors.

Epididymitis

Epididymitis is inflammation of the epididymis. It is usually secondary to orchitis. The organisms cause perivascular lesions with oedema and fibrosis, resulting in epididymal obstruction stasis of epididymal contents and extravasation (flowing out fluid from vessel) of semen. The high lipid and mycolic acid contents lead to the formation of spermatic granuloma.

The diagnosis is based on clinical palpation of the epididymitis to detect enlargement, induration and spermatic granuloma. These lesions are observed in the tail region of the epididymis.

The prognosis is severe or poor even in moderate cases of epididymitis,because obstruction prevents discharge of spermatozoa from testes. In valuable animals with unilateral epididymitis unilateral castration may be performed provided accessory glands and vas deferens have no lesions. Such animals may be given long sexual rest.

Spermiostasis

Spermiostasis may be caused by blind rudimentary mesonephric tubules or ductuli aberrantes. These are most often defective efferent tubules. These defective tubules are attached to rete or epididymis and produce lesions mainly in the head of epididymis. Other portions of the epididymis are only rarely involved. The condition is common in bucks and rams, less common in bulls and rare in other domestic animals. The condition is probably genetic in origin. There is no treatment for this condition and because of hereditary nature of this condition, the affected animals should be culled.

Segmental Aplasia of the Mesonephric Duct

Segmental aplasia of the mesonephric duct is a congenital hereditary condition. The body and tail or all the epididymis and even the part of the vas deferens may be missing. In majority of the cases, the condition is unilateral and the buck is fertile. The bilateral cases are sterile and the semen is watery with no sperm. There is no treatment and the affected animals should not be used in breeding programme as the condition is hereditary.

Pathology of the Vas Deferens and Ampulla

Infections and inflammations of the vas deferens are usually associated with orchitis, epididymis or seminal vasculitis. Usually, the infections are unilateral but may be bilateral. Several infectious organisms e.g. *Brucella abortus, Streptococci, C. pyogenes* and others including viruses may be responsible for this conditions.

Ampullitis is revealed as thickened, firm and painful enlargement. In ampullitis, the semen contains pus cells and the motility of the spermatozoa is poor. If the motility is good after ejaculation, it would be lost rapidly on storage of semen.

Seminal Vesiculitis

Inflammations of the vesicular glands, which lie just lateral to the ampullae of the vas deferens, are commonly seen. Their normal consistency is neat, yielding and lobulations are very clearly felt in normal condition.

The incidence has been reported varying from 3 to 4 percent in European breeds. Some cases are also reported in India.

Seminal vasculitis may be caused by a variety of organisms including specific pathogens (like *Brucella* organisms, *Mycobacterium bovis, Mycobacterium paratuberculosis, Chlamydia, Mycoplasma actinobacilli, Coryneabacteria* etc.) The organisms may localize in the seminal vesicle from other infected foci like rumenitis, liver abscesses and traumatic gastritis. Infections in the seminal vesicle may also come as an ascending infection (e.g. from prepuce) or as a descending infections (e.g. from infected ampulla, epidymis, vas deferens and testicle). In countries where brucellosis is present, Brucella abortus is the most common cause for seminal vesiculitis.

The seminal vesiculitis may be acute or chronic. In acute seminar vesiculitis there would be signs of localized peritonitis. Affected gland (s) may be enlarged and firm and there is pain on palpation. Purulent exudate is present in the semen consistently. Chronic seminal vesiculitis may or may not follow acute phase. There would be enlargement, fibrosis and loss of lobulations from the gland. Pain on palpation is usually absent. In both the forms, semen or affected bulls contains purulent material, leukocytes and epithelial cells and the motility of the sperms is decreased.

The prognosis in seminal vesiculitis may be fair to poor depending upon duration and severity of the infection, nature of infection and the presence of other infected foci. Males affected with brucellosis, tuberculosis mycoplasmosis and with lesions of testes epididymides, ampullae or prostate should be slaughtered.

10

Good Management Practices for Improving Reproductive Efficiency in Goats

R. Pourouchottamane[1], N. Ramachandran[2], Chetna Gangwar[1] and B. Rai[1]

[1]Division of AP&R, ICAR-Central Institute for Research on Goats Makhdoom, Farah, Mathura- 281 122, Uttar Pradesh
[2]Division of Bioenergetics and Environmental Sciences, ICAR- National Institute of Animal Nutrition and Physiology- 560030, Adugodi Bengaluru, Karnataka

India has rich diversity of goat genetic resources and as per 20th livestock census (2019), there are 148.88 million goats in India. They are mostly found in arid and semi-arid regions of the country and one of the mainstay of dryland agriculture system. Out of 148.88 million, around half of them (75 to 60 million goats) are found in Rajasthan (20.84 m), Uttar Pradesh (14.48 m), Madhya Pradesh (11.06 m), Maharashtra (10.6 m), Tamil Nadu (9.89 m) Karnataka (6.17 m) and Gujarat (4.66 m). Out of total goat population, only 35 % of the goats are of either pure breed or upgraded nature resembling the some of the local breeds. There is huge scope to improve the productivity through use of assisted reproductive tools like artificial insemination and estrus synchronization in field condition to upgrade the non-descript population in relatively shorter period of time as compared to natural services.

However, the overall Production and Reproduction efficiency in any species is controlled by multifaceted factors (both genetic and numerous environmental factors) which individually as well as collectively affects the productive and reproductive efficiency of goats ultimately affecting the returns and profitability of the farm. In this Chapter, we will discuss about some of the good management practices (GMPs) to be followed at different stages (birth of the kid to adult stage) including bio-security measures in goat farm for effectively and efficiently harnessing the full genetic potential of the goats. The various factors affecting the goat farming includes

1. GMPs for different age groups of goats including breeding practices/ reproductive management, feeding practices, shelter practices and general care and management.
2. Farm organization and Bio security measures
3. Record keeping

GMPs for different age groups of goats

a. Care and management of New born kids and up to 3 months of age

Female goats about to deliver can be easily identified as their udder is distended with milk and external genital flushed and in flaccid condition. Usually, normal delivery happens in multiparous goats and special care is needed only for goats kidding first time or those being inseminated with semen from larger breeds/ crossed with larger breeds as problem of dystocia may arise.

- The mother generally licks the new born and within minutes, young ones stand on their legs and seek teats for suckling.
- Help the kids which couldn't stand on their own and feed them the colostrum.
- Clean nostrils and body of new-born properly with clean cloth, cut the naval card one inch away from body of new-born and apply diluted tincture iodine solution.
- The new born should be protected from cold, wind and rain as surface area of newborn kids are larger and the kids will lose its body heat quickly and succumb especially in winter season.
- To protect against the inclement weather, the kidding pens should be covered with sheets of thatching material, gunny bags and Tripal.
- During first one week, kids should be housed along with mother in kidding cage (5x5 foot), floor bedded with straw round the clock and allowed free suckling.
- In high yielding does, restrict excess milk consumption by kids using udder bags. The kids born as multiple are usually with lower body weight and weak, therefore assistance needs to be given during suckling.
- Plan for milk replacer or assisted suckling of kids born from low milk producing goats with goats having more milk.
- After one week of age, segregate all the kids and house them together in larger enclosure (10 ft x 10 ft) which can house space around 20-25 kids.

- For the first fortnight, the kids should have access to suckling three times in a day. Later reduce the suckling twice a day.
- After 15-20 days of birth, kids should be offered tender tree fodder leaves along with crushed grains in the shed up to weaning at 3 months of age.
- Up to 3 months of age, temporary identification may be done using neck bands or colour marking
- Weighing should be done at weekly interval up to one month of age, at 15 days interval during one to three months of age so that any issues can be sorted out and also find whether the kids are growing as per its breed specifications.

b. Care and management of kids from 3 months of age

Young ones should not be allowed for grazing for first two to three months and at three-month age the kids are weaned and male and female kids are separated.

- Permanent identification through ear tattooing or ear tagging should be done by three months of age
- Kids should be housed as per their age group and should not be mixed with adult stock. Normally kids are playful; hence sufficient space should be there for movement.
- The extra care should be given as this period is very critical (weaning stress) as well as kids may pick up infection from soil (coccidiosis) and susceptible to respiratory problems like pneumonia.
- Surplus male kids having lower weight gain/growth may be castrated at 2-3 months of age and used for fattening while kids showing faster growth and progeny of high yielding dam may be retained for future breeding.
- Growing kid should be given adequate concentrate and fodder for proper growth and early sexual maturity.
- Growing animals should be housed as per age group. i.e., 3 to 6 months, 6 to 9 months and 9 to 12 months of age.
- The floor space requirement of goats of different age groups are given below

Age of goats/ Sheep	Covered area (m^2/sq.ft)	Open paddock (m^2/sq.ft)
0 to 3 months	0.2-0.25/2.5	0.4-0.5 /5.0
3-6 months	0.5-0.75 /5-7.5	1.0-1.5 /10-15
6-12 months	0.75-1.0 /7.5-10	1.5-2.0 /2.5
Yearling goats (12-24 months)	1.0 /10	2.0 /20.0
Adult Goats (1-3 Years)	1.5 /15	3.0 /30
Pregnant and lactating goats	1.5-2.0 /15-20	3.0-4.0 /30-40
Bucks	1.5-2.0 /15-20	3.0-4.0 /30-40

c. Selection of Male and Female adult goats for breeding

Female: Females around one year of age in medium sized breed and 15 months of age in large sized breed should be used for breeding purpose. Breeding too young female will hinder its own growth as well as results in difficult birth and higher kid loss. Females selected for breeding should have breed characters, i.e., pure bred. The females from does which are high yielder should be invariably included in the breeding stock. Similarly, the females having poor milking capacity and physical deformities should be removed from breeding flock. The selected female should have been voluminous, symmetrical udder with medium sized teats. Angular hind legs with wide roomy hind quarters will provide good space between inner aspects of thighs for development of voluminous udder.

Male: Males selected for breeding purpose should be true to its breed character in terms of morphology and physical conformation. Buck should be in good body condition (feed extra concentrate during breeding season to maintain its body condition), muscular and strong legs with normal gait. It should have two well-developed testicles and should show good libido. Breeding buck should be in good body condition, masculine and legs should be stronger with normal gait. As selected male for breeding is contributing genetic material for half of the future flock, the selection of male animals should be stringent, Male's mother should be high milk producer and there should be no genetic defects in both parents. Male kids showing higher body weight gain during growing stage as well as those born as twins should be retained for future use as breeding bucks.

d. Reproductive/ Breeding management tips

- **Choose breed** (especially while going for artificial insemination) according to **adaptability for prevailing climatic conditions**, purpose of rearing and suitability for feeding management system.

- Many local breeds are having valuable adaptive traits that have developed over a long period of time which includes tolerance to extreme climates, diseases and adaptability to survive, regularly produce and reproduce in low input management conditions and feeding regimes.
- Local climate resilient breeds of moderate productivity should be promoted over susceptible crossbreds. For example, Performance and survivability of goat breeds of North-western region deteriorate in hot and humid eastern regions/ western ghat regions. The semen from these local climate resilient breeds may be used for artificial insemination for upgrading the non-descript goats of their tract and adjoining regions. (Table no.)

State/ region	**Goat breeds available**
Gujarat	Surti, Zalawadi, Gohilwadi, Kutchi, Mehsana and Kahmi
Rajasthan	Jakhrana, Sirohi, Sojat, Karuli, Gujari and Marwari
Maharashtra	Sangamneri, Osmanabadi, Berari and Konkan Kanyal
Tamil Nadu	Kodi-Adu, Kanni-Adu and Salem-black
Uttar Pradesh	Jamunapari, Barbari and Rohil Khandi
Madhya Pradesh	Jamunapari, Bundhelkhandi
Kerala	Malabari and Attapady Black
Karnataka	Bidri and Nandidurga
Himachal Pradesh, J & K	Chegu, Changthangi, Gaddi and Bhakarwali
Punjab	Beetal
Orissa	Ganjam
Uttarakhand	Pantja
West Bengal, Bihar,Jharkhand	Black Bengal
Assam	Assam Hill
Nagaland	Sumi-Ne
A & N Island	Teressa

Breeding bucks in the flock should be replaced once in 2 to 3 years to avoid inbreeding.

- Females may be bred during April-May and during October-November months so that kids will be born in favourable environment (avoiding extreme hot or cold season). Female showing signs of heat in morning need to be mated during evening and vice versa (10 to 14 hours after signs of estrus begin).
- Females may be provided with flushing (additional 100 to 200gm. concentrate) ration 15 days before breeding which will increase the chances of multiple births.

- Similarly, females in last trimester of pregnancy may be given steaming up ration so that body condition of mother will improve which results in higher milk yield and higher birth weight of kids.
- Regular culling of low performing male and females is prerequisite in any farm for improving the genetic merit of the flock as well as improving the profitability of the farm.

e. Care of pregnant goat

- Separate the females in advanced stage of pregnancy from the flock and effective care should be taken in their feeding (steaming up ration). The pregnant does should not be handled frequently.
- Provide adequate nutrition, easily digestible and laxative diet. Extra feeding during the latter part of pregnancy (3-4 weeks before parturition) will be beneficial for the body conditioning of goats (positive energy balance) which will help in improving milk production and higher birth weight of kids.
- Do not allow them to fight with each other and do not allow them to mix with recently aborted animals.
- Does in advanced stage of pregnancy should be kept in a separate shed 4-6 days before partition and maximum comfort like soft clean bedding and individual kidding pen should be provided.
- Shortly before the doe is due to kid, clip hair around the udder, hind quarters and tail for greater cleanliness. Does should be protected from chilly weather condition.

Prophylactic Measures in Organized Farm

The general preventive measures include following proper vaccination against important infectious diseases, deworming and dipping to prevent endo and ectoparasitic loads in the herd, quarantine of newly bought animals, isolation facility for separating sick animals and proper disposal of dead animals.

Hygiene and sanitization are first and foremost aspect to prevent spreadof diseases.

- Unwanted entry into the farm to be restricted
- Foot Bath at entry point of the farm is mandatory and width of the foot bath should be so wide so that no one can jump over it and so deep that sole of the shoes gets dipped and disinfected. Add $KMnO_4$ tablets or copper sulphate powder to the water in foot bath.

- Daily cleaning of the surroundings of the farm and inside of the sheds
- Applying of Lime powder inside the shed once in a week if there is dampness and to avoid spread of diseases
- Changing the soil inside the shed once in a year (it will reduce the burden of infections built in the soil due to dung, urine etc)
- Strict biosecurity measures (No new animal to be entered into farm without quarantine period of 21 to 28 days)
- The sick animals should be separated, and treated in the isolation ward till recovery. Dead animals should be removed immediately, and should be disposed by burning or deep burial.
- Entry of stray animals such as dogs, cats, wild animals etc. should be strictly prohibited.
- Any protruding structure or object which may cause injury to animals, should be removed immediately from the farm.
- Animals should be prevented from entering water logged areas where chances of occurrence of foot diseases are more. Trimming of hooves should be done at least four times in a year.
- The farm activities (vaccination, deworming, dipping, drenching, screening, quarantine etc.) should be practiced as per the standard recommendations.

Vaccination: Goats are vulnerable to infectious diseases and it requires timely vaccination. A vaccination schedule or calendar has to be prepared to plan and execute the vaccination in time for the herd.

Deworming Parasites, mainly internal parasites are one of the biggest problems of organized goat farming. In addition to significant morbidity and mortality, the parasites contribute to the poor growth and unthriftiness in the goats. Hence, deworming is necessary in goats to prevent the infections caused by the endoparasites. In case of organized goat farms, deworming is done twice in a year: pre-rainy season and post-rainy season.

Drenching is applied to prevent coccidiosis in goats, and is done between 1 to 6 months of age because coccidiosis is generally seen during the age mentioned.

Dipping: It is done to prevent infestations caused by ectoparasites and is applied before and after winter season.

Quarantine of new bought animals

Whenever, new animals are need to be added in the flock, they should be kept separately away from the farm animals and needs to be observed for 4 to 6 weeks period for presence of any diseases. During this period, complete vaccination, deworming, dipping, drenching before merging these new animals into the farm.

Regular Screening of animals

The regular screening of animals in the farm is utmost important in maintaining the productivity of the herd. Before breeding season, all breeding animals especially, males should be screened for brucellosis at six-month interval and all the positive animals must be culled immediately.

Culling: At organized goat farm, culling is an ongoing process which never ends. The purpose of culling is to dispose of unproductive goats from the farm to save unnecessary maintenance expenditure on unproductive animals. There are mainly two grounds for culling of animals i.e., culling on production ground and culling on health ground.

Importance of Record Keeping

Record keeping on pedigree, breeding, production, reproduction, health traits in the goat farm is essential for bringing genetic improvement in flock. Identification (tagging/ tattooing) of goat is prerequisite for record keeping and selection of animals. A record keeping must be simple, have accurate data that is useful and which can easily be converted into information, and must be easily retrievable to make informed Decisions

Simplified formats of Records

The simplified format of different records to be used under field conditions by the farmers is given here under:

Breeding Register

S.No.	Animal Number	Date of Birth	Sire No.	Dam No.	Date of Service	Date of kidding	Type of Kidding	Number of kids	Sex of kids	Abnormality if any
1										
2										
3										
4										

Kidding Register

S. No.	Animal No	Sire No	Dam No	Sex	Type of Birth	Date of Birth	Remarks
1							
2							
3							
4							

Body Weight/ Growth Register

S.No.	AnimalNo	Date of Birth	Sire No	Dam No	Type of Birth	Sex	Birth weight	1 month weight.	2 month weight	3 month weight	6 month weight	9 month weight	12 month weight	Remarks (Sold/ Died)
1														
2														
3														
4														
5														

Sale Register

S.No.	Animal No.	Date of Sale	Sex of animal	Age of animal	Weight of animal	Rate of the animal	To whomsold	Sold for Breeding/ Sacrifice/ Meat purpose
1								
2								
3								
4								
5								

Treatment and Mortality Register

S.No.	Animal No.	Date of Illness	Particulars	Date of Recovery	Remarks, if Died, Date
1					
2					
3					
4					
5					

Annual Preventive Health Care Register

S.No.	Particulars	Date	Remarks
	Vaccination		
1	FMD vaccine First Dose		
2	FMD vaccine Second dose after six months		
3	H S vaccine		
4	Goat Pox		
5	ET Vaccine		
6	ET Vaccine (Booster)		
7	PPR (once in three years)		
	Deworming of flock (Three monthly interval)		
8	First		
9	Second		
10	Third		
11	Fourth		
	Ectoparasite control of flock (half yearly interval)		
12	First		
13	Second		

Thus, with proper recording of the events in the farm, the goat farm owner can easily keep track of events like:

- Whether activities are going according to plan,
- Whether yields and profits are improving or going down,
- When animals were vaccinated, dipped, given any medicine or castrated etc.

- Keep track of assets: Progress in the farm operation cannot be determined from year to year without keeping an inventory.

Further, records are the important tool for selection of breeding animals and bringing overall genetic improvement in the farm thereby increasing the profitability.

11

Sexual Behaviour in Buck

Chetna Gangwar and R. Pourouchottamane

Division of AP&R, ICAR-Central Institute for Research on Goats, Makhdoom Mathura- 281 122, Uttar Pradesh

The animals are mostly social ones and prefer living in herds. In each species there are certain rules for group survival, cohesion, defence and also for propagation. The basic patterns of male sexual behaviour appear to be innate in nature. Kids of both sexes are very often seen exhibiting sexual display during play and mounting is seen most commonly. In females the sexual receptivity is restricted to few hours or days near the estrous phase of the estrous cycle, while in males the sexual receptivity is grossly permanent. The physiological signals for arousal of sexual motivations originate from gonadal steroid balance. However, the secretion of gonadal steroids is not permanent. In males the androgen secretion is in the form of several peaks within 24 hours reflecting the pulsatile release of pituitary gonadotropins. However, the total amount of androgen in males is almost constant practically for day to day. In females the secretions of estrogens are restricted only during few days (follicular phase) of the estrous cycle.

The various components of copulatory patterns in male domestic animals are:

1. Sexual arousal
2. Courtship (sexual display)
3. Erection
4. Penile protrusion
5. Mounting
6. Intromission
7. Ejaculation
8. Dismounting
9. Refractoriness

Each response becomes a stimulus for next component of the copulatory pattern. The event of courtship and copulation are shorter in bucks (few second or so) and are longer in swine (about 5 minutes or even more) and horse (about 40 seconds).

Sexual arousal: The finding of the sexual partner is the first step for sexual arousal and in that all the senses like sight, hearing and olfaction are important. The senses of sight, hearing and olfaction help estrous females to be attracted towards the males. The stimuli from males greatly influence the females for exhibiting sexual responses.

Courtship (sexual display): The patterns of courtship are simple in domestic animals but species- specific differences do occur. Once attracted to a female partner, the buck tests her receptivity most oftenly by sniffing and licking around the perineal region. These actions indicate chemical communication in between the male and female partners. Sniffing to female's genitalia and urine is very common in goat. Following sniffing of female's genitalia and urine, the male stands rigidly, makes the head in horizontal position with neck extended and the upper lips are curled upward to perform the "Flehmens reaction". Characteristic odour does not appear to play a role during courtship. However, species specific patterns of urination during courtship are noticed in some species. There is rhythmic emission of urine during sexual activity in goats, frequent miction on forelegs is seen during sexual activity.

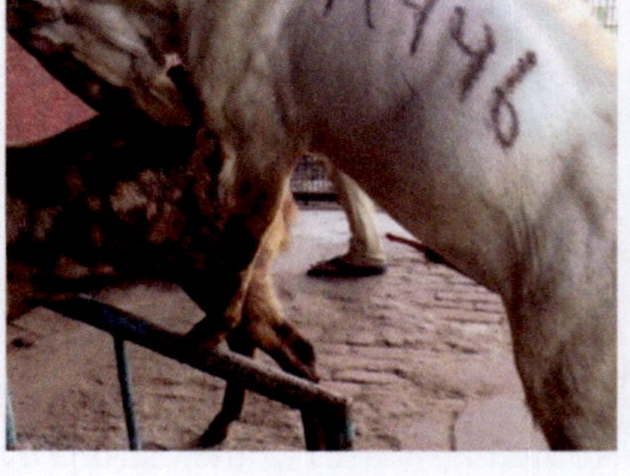

Vocalization species specific vocalization patterns are also observed in males during courtship. Courting bleats are noticed in male goat during sexual display.

Nudging (nudge =to push gently specially to draw attention) and licking of the female's external genitalia and perineal region are notice in goat. Nudging of the female through forelegs is commonly seen in sheep and goat.

The penis of the sexually active male may erect partially and there may be to and fro penile movements before mounting. The male rests his chin on female's body and the receptive female respond by standing quietly in order to allow mounting by the male.

Mounting: During this process the movements of buck's hind limbs and contractions of his abdominal muscles particularly the rectus abdominis muscle align the glans penis both horizontally and vertically to seek vulva for penetration. The male mounts, grasps the female by fixing fore legs around female's body. During this process rhythmic pelvic thrusts may be performed.

Intromission: In farm animals one intromission takes place per copulation. At mounting, the male's pelvic region is brought in close apposition to the female's external genitalia. The movements of the male help the glans penis to seek vulva. The vulvar heat and moisture are detected by the superficial nerve endings of the glans penis and this sensation is the leading factor for proper intromission. The intromission is instant in buck.

Ejaculation: Generalized muscular contractions especially of abdominal muscles take place at ejaculation. The process of ejaculation starts from epididymis, travel along ductus deferens and at the same time accessory sex glands contract and their contents are forced into urethra. Oxytocin is released and causes transport of semen in the epididymis and ductus deference. Rhythmic contractions of the urethral, ischiocavernosus and bulbocavernosus muscles cause release of semen from urethra. At ejaculation, there is maximum lengthening of the penis so that the semen is ejaculated near os cervix in case of goat. At ejaculation in sheep and goat, the male's head is suddenly moved backward.

Dismounting: After the ejaculation has taken place the male dismounts and soon the penis is withdrawn in to the prepuce. Postcoital displays are rare in domestic animals but the male goat licks the penis after ejaculation.

Refractoriness: Most of the males would not show sexual interest in females immediately following copulation and this is known as refractoriness. The period of refractoriness varies greatly in between individual males. Repeated and successive copulations greatly increase the period of refractoriness. The period of refractoriness is modified by environmental stimuli e.g., male to female ratio, cyclicity of the female, length of the breeding season and social interaction among animals. The presentation of new stimuli can revitalize sexual interest in males. Generally, the approach of the male towards the female is selective in nature. The goat reaches exhaustion after a smaller number of ejaculations than ram and bull. After long period of sexual rest, a buck may perform up to 50 services during the breeding season.

12

Semen Collection from Bucks

Chetna Gangwar, Ravi Ranjan and Manish Kumar

Division of AP&R, ICAR-Central Institute for Research on Goats Makhdoom, Mathura- 281 122, Uttar Pradesh

---

Hygienic collection of semen is an integral part of the artificial insemination process. Semen collection implies mounting a teaser doe or a dummy. Therefore, proper semen collection deserves the utmost attention. Sexual efficiency is measured by the percentage or successful semen collections among attempted collections. When males are allowed to female teaser, the male exhibits characteristic behavioural symptoms such as sniffing, nudging or mounting at that time it is necessary for the operator to attempt an approach. This approach has to be done quietly to avoid a fear reflex in the male. The male, even if it mounts the female, deviation of its penis into the receptacle. Under the circumstances, the operator should not more from his squatting position, so that the male does not associate the two events. The animal generally comes back by itself to attempt remounting the female and will serve the artificial vagina. The operator should also stimulate the male by voice.

Points to be remember for semen collection

1. The best time of semen collection is early morning before feeding and in morning hours bucks are fresh and alert.
2. Bucks may reluctant to donate semen in full belly after feeding.
3. If semen is collected early in a day, it can be utilized the same day by liquid semen insemination and this may help in achieving higher fertility.
4. The buck prior to semen collection should be properly cleaned and it is essential to clear the abdominal area, forward and around the sheaths.
5. It is very difficult to collect semen completely free from microorganisms even under strict hygienic conditions but washing of preputial sheath with 0.9% sterile saline solution, 20 minutes prior to semen collection significantly reduces the bacterial load in semen.

6. Artificial Vagina, Liner, collection cups, water etc. should be properly sterilized tomaintain the semen quality.

Organization of the Collecting pens

All the males required for semen are brought into one or two collecting pens made of iron cages. A collecting pen of 8"x8" may be sufficient to collect 6-8 bucks depending on the breed and size. There should be sufficient space for mobility. The collecting pen should be nearer to the laboratory where the processing of semen has to be done, so that after collection, it takes minimum time for evaluation. The dummy is then immobilized in a collection crate.

Artificial vagina (AV) and electro-ejaculator (E.E.) are the two methods for semen collection in bucks. AV method is being used as universal method for routine semen collection.

1. Electro-ejaculator (E.E.)

The Electro-ejaculation method is rarely used for semen collection in bucks. This method is painful to bucks and is generally used for collecting semen from untrained, crippled and valuable sires incapable of service and also in old bucks which have no desire to mount. In this method, weak, alternating current is provided to sacral pelvic nerves with electrode placed in the rectum. This method is comparatively time consuming and required more technical skill. Excessive stimulation at higher voltage may cause a degree of ataxia or the buck may fall down.

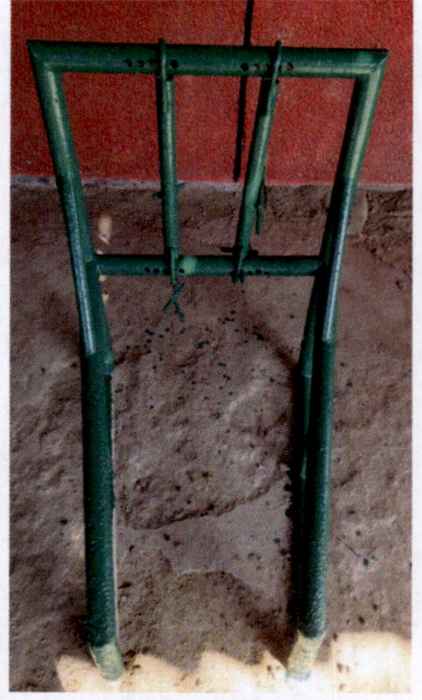

2. The Artificial Vagina Method

This is most common method of semen collection in bucks. Through AV a complete and clean ejaculate is promptly obtained.

Materials required for semen collection

i. **Goat Treves:** It is required to fix the estrus doe so that buck can easily mount on the doe.

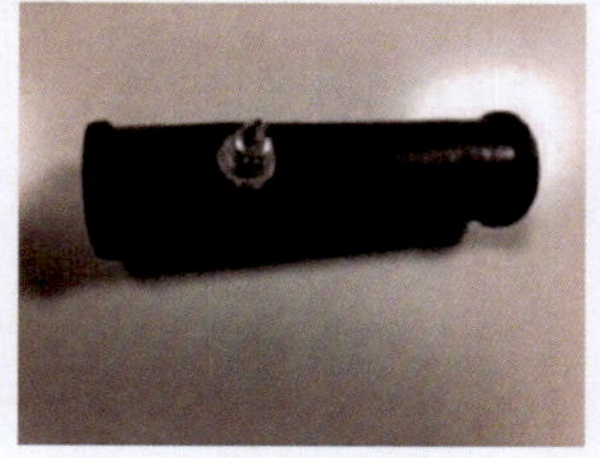

ii. **Estrus doe:** It is better to use estrus doe for semen collection because it enhances the libido as well as quality/quantity of semen ejaculate.

iii. **Artificial vagina**: The semen from buck can be successfully collected by Danish type of AV using an anestrus or estrus doe as dummy. Artificial vagina for goat is made of heavy rubber with 20 cm length and 5 cm diameter as designed by Milovanovic which was later on modified by Rath.

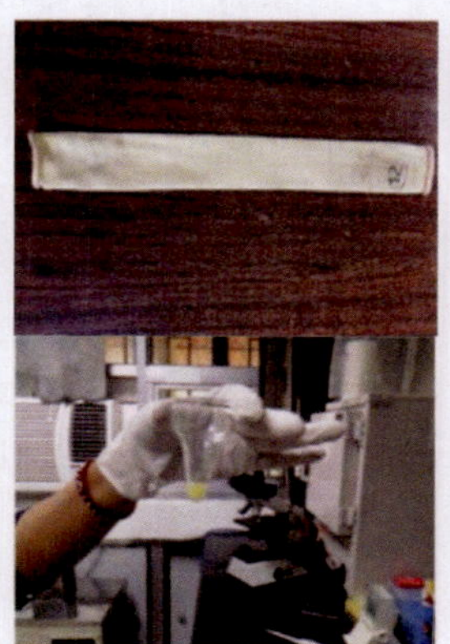

iv. **Rubber liner:** A rubber lining of 30 cm length and 5 cm diameter is inserted in the AV and ends are folded back over the AV.

v. **Semen collection cups**: A graduated glass semen collection cup with measuring efficiency of 0.1 ml should be used for semen collection.

vi. **Hot water:** AV is three-fourths filled with warm water (44-48ºC) and the quantity of water to be filled inside should be 150-175 ml; the temperature of AV ready for use should be around 39ºC.

vii. **Liquid paraffin:** One end (opposite to the valve) of the AV should be lubricated with liquid paraffin so that during intromission penis of the buck may not be injured.

Preparation of Artificial Vagina (AV)

Artificial Vagina (AV) is the most commonly accepted method for semen collection of bulls, buffalo bulls, bucks, horses etc. Artificial Vagina suited and designed for different animal species are commercially available. AV is three-fourths filled with warm water (44-48ºC) and the air is then blown in through the valve to adjust the pressure, so that finally the shape becomes similar to that of natural one. The quantity of water to be filled inside should be 150-175 ml; the temperature of AV ready for use should be around 39ºC. Proper pressure of the AV is also important to stimulate ejaculatory response. Pressure is maintained by inflating air through the vent till such time that the thumb may easily be inserted into the lumen of the AV A graduated glass semen collection cup is held at one end (nearer to valve) of AV and the other end is lubricated with the soft paraffin to avoid injury to buck due to friction. Now, AV is ready to collect the semen.

Steps in semen collection

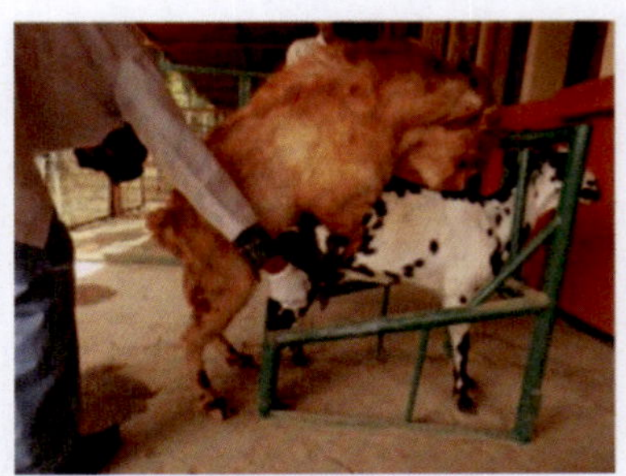

1. Secure dummy in a Treves.
2. The operator should sit preferably right side of the dummy with AV ready in one hand.
3. The buck is allowed one or two false mounts until it is noted at what stage of mounting the penis thrushes forward.
4. On the next mount, the operator advances the artificial vagina towards the end of the penis; the penis is deflected into AV, so that a single thrust will result in ejaculation. It is necessary to take care in placing the artificial vagina in prolongation of the penis in order to ensure complete penetration of the artificial vagina.
5. Immediately after ejaculation, the male dismounts, and the AV is held vertically, in order to permit descent of the ejaculate in the lower part of the collection cup where graduations are engraved. Soon after collection, the semen should be delivered to the laboratory for evaluation.
6. The semen collection cup is withdrawn from the AV This is kept well protected from light and temperature shock. It is marked for identification, corked or covered and is put in a water bath at 35-37°C.

13

Buck Semen Dilution for Cryopreservation

Chetna Gangwar, Ravi Ranjan and Manish Kumar

Division of AP&R, ICAR-Central Institute for Research on Goats Makhdoom Mathura- 281 122, Uttar Pradesh

---

Why we do semen dilution?

The following objectives are accomplished by semen dilution/ extension

- Preservation of semen potential over a long period of time.
- Increase in the number of services per ejaculate. Ideally approximately 40 does can be inseminated from diluted/ extended semen of a single ejaculate.
- Extenders provide the spermatozoa with a medium in which they are able to remain viable and fertile for a prolonged time period. An ideal extender should be able to provide a conducive environment to facilitate sperm survival and modify the sperm structure to prepare them for freezing through the following properties:
- It should be isotonic with blood and should maintain this during preservation.
- It should have capacity of maintenance of pH (6.6-6.8) with high buffering capacity in that range.
- It should ensure supply of metabolites for nutrition and survival of sperm cells.
- It should contain lipoprotein and lecithin, minerals in adequate quantity and should contain substances to be used for aerobic metabolism by spermatozoa.
- It should provide protection against cryoinjuries.
- It should prevent the formation of ice crystals.

- It should not contain any material which may exert any adverse effect on spermatozoa, female genitalia, fertilization process or growth and development of the zygote.
- It should contain antibiotic in sufficient quantity to check the microbial growth.

Preparation of TRIS- citric acid-egg yolk glycerol extender and Processingof Semen for Cryopreservation

The Tris-citric acid-egg yolk glycerol extender is the most frequently used extender in the cryopreservation of cattle and buffalo semen. Preparation of the extender plays a very important role in determining the quality of the processed semen. Therefore, care must be taken to ensure that the extender is prepared aseptically and it contains all the ingredients in appropriate concentration. Extender should always be prepared under a laminar air flow. It is also important to check that the pH and osmolarity of the semen extender for a particular species corresponds to the prescribed limits for that particular species. The tris, citric acid, fructose, egg yolk and glycerol contains the following ingredients:

Protective agent: Egg yolk, glycerol

Sugar: Fructose

Antibiotics: Penicillin and streptomycin

Buffer: TRIS (tris-hydroxymethyl amino methane)-citric acid monohydrate

Cryoprotective Action of Glycerol

Glycerol exerts cryoprotective effect by the following ways:

- It binds with water and decreases the freezing point of the solution and acts through 'salt buffering mechanism.
- It inhibits lactic acid production and prolongs sperm survival
- It enters the sperm cell and binds some of the intracellular water and protects sperm from mechanical damage by intracellular as well as extracellular water crystal formation and changes in concentration of electrolytes.

Method of Preparation of TRIS-citric acid-egg yolk-glycerol Extender

Solution A

TRIS 3.06 g

Citric acid monohydrate 1.65g

Glycerol 6.00 ml

Fructose (anhydrous) 1.00g

Triple glass distilled water upto 100 ml

This solution is sterilized by autoclaving at 15 psi for 20 minute sprior to fructose addition.

Add Benzyl Penicillin Sodium (1 Lakh IU) and Streptomycin sulphate (100 mg) to prepare TRIS buffer. This buffer can be stored at 4°C for 3-4 days.

TRIS Extender

TRIS extender is prepared by adding 10% egg yolk to Tris buffer. This should be prepared fresh at the time of use and thoroughly mixed using magnetic stirrer. It should be maintained at 34°C at the time of semen processing.

Extender composition

Preparation of TRIS buffer

Ingredients	**Quantity**
TRIS buffer (Tris hydroxymethyl) aminomethane 2- Amino-2-(hydroxymethyl) propane-1, 3- diol	3.06 gm
Citric acid (monohydrate)	1.65gm
Fructose (anhydrous)	1.0 gm
Penicillin G. Sodium	60 mg
Di hydro streptomycin sulfate	100 mg
Glycerol	6 ml
Egg yolk	10 ml
Double glass distilled water	up to 100 ml

Preparation of Egg Yolk

Egg yolk is prepared from fresh hen's egg procured from a known source or farm which is free from infection. Procurement of egg from market should be avoided as there are chances of microbial contamination. Eggs should not be stored for more than 2-3 days at 4°C. Eggs should never be cleaned by washing with water as there is chance of influx of water/ contaminant through porous egg shell. It should be wiped clean with 70% alcohol before storage and before breaking it.

The forceps and hands should be wiped clean with 70% alcohol before breaking the egg. The egg should be broken into two halves and the white of the egg should be drained into a beaker. The yolk is transferred to a clean and sterilized filter paper and rolled over the filter paper so as to remove the white. The yolk membrane is then punctured by sterile straw / needle to drain yolk in a sterile measuring cylinder. Required quantity of yolk is prepared for reconstitution of the diluents.

Dilution rate

The semen is extended to such an appropriate volume so that each inseminating dose of semen contains sufficient number of motile spermatozoa needed for optimum fertility. The following should be ensured before dilution

i) All sterilized glass wares and other articles are assembled on the working bench in advance.

ii) Semen and dilutor are maintained at equal temperature.

Calculation of dilution rate

Volume of ejaculate = 1ml

Density/ml = 4000×10^6

Motile spermatozoa 70%

1ml of semen contains $\dfrac{4000 \times 10^6 \times 70}{100}$

$= 2800 \times 10^6$ motile sperms

For semen cryopreservation 1 ml diluted semen must contain 400×10^6 motile sperms

Hence the dilution rate is $\dfrac{2800 \times 10^6}{400 \times 10^6} = 7$

Hence 1 ml of the semen may be diluted to $1 \times 7 = 7$ ml

Procedure of dilution

As a precaution, small quantity of the dilutor may be added slowly to the few drops of the semen. If this is maintained satisfactorily, the whole semen may be extended. They would save the semen; in case the dilutor is not fit for sperm survival due to any mistake at any step. After initial checking the dilution of the semen should be done in two steps. The first step dilution is done immediately after semen collection and its initial examination. The second step (final) dilution should be done after detailed semen examination and assessing the final dilution rate so that each dose of insemination contains minimum number of normal and motile spermatozoa for optimum fertility.

14

Semen Evaluation by Traditional Methods

Chetna Gangwar and Manish Kumar

Division of AP&R, ICAR-Central Institute for Research on Goats Makhdoom, Mathura- 281 122, Uttar Pradesh

The semen evaluation is of great importance in predicting fertility of the male. There are several parameters to evaluate the semen quality. Usually bucks with good semen samples have good fertility and bucks with poor or very poor semen samples are invariably infertile or sterile. A single test is never sufficient to assess the semen quality and the examiner should be acquainted with several tests to evaluate the semen. The semen should be examined with in a shortest possible period after ejaculation and the ejaculate must be properly protected and handled until examination. Semen can be evaluated by following methods

i) Macroscopic test

ii) Microscopic test

iii) Metabolic test

Macroscopic test

These tests can be performed by visual examination of the semen.

A) **Appearance:** Semen with curdy appearance indicate reproductive infections. Translucent samples contain few spermatozoa. Uniform and opaque appearance of the ejaculate is indicative of high spermatozoa concentration.

B) **Colour:** The colour of buck semen can be milky, creamy or yellowish due to the presence of a harmless pigment "Riboflavin" secreted by the accessory glands. Buck with orchitis may donate semen of brownish colour because of blood pigment. Dark red or bloody semen is indicative of blood which may come from tubular genital tract. Clots or flakes in the semen may be due to the pus that may come from tubular tract or accessory glands. Semen may of greenish yellow in colour due to the presence of *Pseudomonas aeruginosa* in it.

C) **Consistency:** By visual examination, the estimation of the sperm concentration may be done fairly satisfactorily. The visual characteristics of buck semen corresponding to spermatozoa density are as below

Visual Consistency	Sperm Concentration/ml
Creamy	2.5×10^6/ ml and above
Light creamy	1.5 to 2.5×10^6
Milky	0.5 to 1.5×10^6
Cloudy-watery	0.1 to 0.5×10^6
Watery	$< 0.1\times 10^6$

D) **Volume:** The semen volume is generally less in young and small sized buck, excessively used bucks, during incomplete ejaculation and bucks with seminal vasculitis. Teasing increases the ejaculate volume. If the low ejaculate volume is accompanied by low spermatozoa concentration, the number of sperm available would also be low and hence would minimize the use of semen. In bucks the average ejaculate volume is 0.5 to 1.5 ml.

Microscopic test

A) Mass Motility

The sperm motility at the time of collection is used as a measure to assess the fertilizing capacity of the sperm. It indicates both the sperm concentration and their viability. For judging mass motility of the spermatozoa, a drop of freshly collected semen is spread uniformly over a clean grease free and dry slide maintained at 35°C and is examined under low power of the microscope with the facility of electrically heated stage to maintain the temperature. The following numerical scales are assigned to different waves/swirls motion as observed under the microscope.

Microscopic findings	Numerical scale	Percentage of motilesperm
Extremely rapid waves and eddies	5	90 % or more
The waves and eddies are comparatively not so rapid	4	80-90
The waves are slowly moving and are scattered in the field	3	50-80
The waves and eddies are absent with movement of spermatozoa	2	40
No waves are observed, only stationary and throbbing movements are observed	1	20
Spermatozoa are non motile	0	0

Sperm Concentration

Sperm concentration is measured to determine the number of spermatozoa per ml of neat semen. There are three methods for determining the sperm concentration:

i) Direct visual assessment of the consistency of the ejaculate:

This technique is practiced in some artificial insemination centers. However, this test is not accurate due to subjective assessment and should not be used in practice.

ii) Haemocytometer technique:

This technique is an accurate technique and more reliable and commonly used.

iii) Calorimetric/spectrophotometric technique:

This is most efficient technique as it involves less time and results are more precise. But, before using the material in routine conditions, it is necessary to obtain a standard curve by using at least 50 samples of known and different concentrations of spermatozoa, previously determined by haemocytometer counting chamber. The sperm concentration varies from 2000 to 5000 million per ml in different breeds of buck. Sperm number per ejaculate is calculated by multiplication of the volume and the sperm concentration.

C) Individual Motility

The estimate of initial mass motility is not a very precise method. Some weakly motile spermatozoa may be exaggerated by surrounding very active spermatozoa. To avoid this, the individual spermatozoa are observed under the microscope to estimate the total percentage of motile sperm cells in the ejaculate. For the estimation of individual spermatozoa motility, the semen is diluted (1:100) in normal saline solution or Ringer's solution. One drop of the diluted semen is put on a clean and dry slide and is covered by cover slip. The slide is examined under high power (40×) in a microscope having warm stage facility.

D) Live and Dead count

Dead spermatozoa could be differentiated by their ability to get stained by Eosin dye. The live spermatozoa, which are alive at the time of staining, remain colourless since they were impermeable to the Eosin stain. Nigrosin provided a blue-black background.

Composition of Eosin-Nigrosin stain

Eosin – Y (Water Soluble)	1.67 gm
Nigrosin (Water Soluble)	10.00 gm
Sodium citrate buffer (2.9%, pH=6.8)	100 ml

Procedure- One small drop of semen sample (kept at 35°C) is mixed with 2 to 3 drops of Eosin-Nigrosin stain on a clean glass slide kept on a thermostatically warm stage (34-35^{0}C). This mixture is kept for 1 min. A smear is then prepared from the mixture on a clean and grease free glass slide. It is dried in air and examined under the bright field 100X oil immersion objective of phase contrast microscope. Around 200 sperms should be assessed. Sperms that are colorless (unstained) are classified as live and those that showed any pink colour are classified as dead. Per cent viable spermatozoa are calculated as

$$\text{Per cent live spermatozoa} = \frac{\text{Viable spermatozoa counted}}{\text{Total spermatozoa counted}} \times 100$$

E) Sperm Abnormalities

The recognition of defective spermatozoa in stained smears provides useful information. The bucks' fertility depends upon morphologically normal spermatozoa present in the ejaculate. The fertility is affected if the abnormal spermatozoa exceed beyond 20%. In good quality semen samples, there should not be a greater number of primary abnormalities like micro cephalic head, macro cephalic head, elongated narrow head, short broad head, pyriform head, double mid piece, highly coiled mid piece, swelling of mid piece, abaxially attached mid piece etc. Eosin-Nigrosin stained slide can be used for counting of abnormalities.

F) Acrosomal Integrity

Giemsa stain is used to assess the acrosomal integrity of frozen thawed buck spermatozoa as per Watson (1975). Diluted semen drop should be kept on clean grease free slide and thin tongue shape smear is prepared. After air drying the smear, the slide is fixed in methanol for 15 min and then after washing the fixed slide is kept in working solution of Giemsa for 90 min. Excess stain is removed by gentle stream of water. It is dried in air and examined under the bright field 100× oil immersion objective of phase contrast microscope. Around 200 sperms must be assessed in different five fields of a slide.

Preparation of Giemsa stock solution

i) Dissolve 1g Giemsa in 66 ml Glycerol in mortal.

ii) Pour the mixed liquid in the flask and heat it on magnetic stirrer on 60° C for one hour.

iii) Cool it at room temperature and add 84 ml of methanol in the flask and mix it.

iv) Stock solution of 150 ml of Giemsa is ready.

Preparation of Giemsa stock solution

It should be prepared just before use.

i) Giemsa stock solution - 3 ml

ii) Sorensen's 0.1 M phosphate buffer - 2ml

iii) Distilled water- 35 ml

G) Hypo-osmotic Swelling Test-

The HOS test is based on swelling ability of functioning sperms after being exposed to hypo-osmotic solution. Fluid is transferred into the cell through plasma membrane of spermatozoa, trying to achieve balance between intracellular and extracellular spaces, and functionally intact membrane begins to swell starting at the tail of spermatozoa. Such spermatozoa are referred as swelled or HOS reactive/positive (HOS+) signifying functionally intact membranes. Spermatozoa with functionally defective membrane do not swell and their tail does not invaginate (Jayendran *et al*., 1984).

Hypo-osmotic solution of 100 mOsmol/L was prepared by dissolving the following reagents in the given concentrations for semen evaluation.

I	Sodium citrate	0.49 gm
II	Fructose	0.90 gm
III	Double distilled water	up to 100 ml

Procedure

One ml of hypo-osmotic solution, having an osmotic strength of 100 mosm/l is mixed with 0.1 ml of semen, and incubated in a water bath at 37^{0}C for one hour. Following incubation, a drop of well mixed solution is taken on a clean dry glass slide and covered with a cover-slip. Sperm tail curling is recorded as an effect of swelling due to influx of water. A total of 200 spermatozoa are counted in different fields at 400x magnification under phase contrast microscope. These spermatozoa are classified in four different classes according to presence of following swelling pattern (Takahashi *et al.,* 1990).

Patterns observed

i. No swelling, no membrane reaction (HOS-)
ii. Swelling of the tip of the tail (HOS+)
iii. Different type of hair pin like swelling or swelling of mid-piece (HOS+)
iv. Complete tail coiling (HOS+)

H) Physio-Chemical test

Following parameters may be examined to evaluate semen e.g. pH, viscosity, osmotic pressure, electrical conductivity and Methylene Blue Reduction test. Out of above test only pH is used in routine practice and for other tests are requires a lot of facilities and is also time consuming.

I) Metabolic test

Some of the metabolic tests are listed below but these tests are more tedious and difficult to conduct at artificial insemination centers. Although some of the tests are correlated with fertility but because of difficulties in conducting these tests at artificial insemination centers it is of less practical utility.

i. Catalase test
ii. Resistance to cold shock
iii. Millovanov's Resistance Test
iv. Methylene blue Reduction Test
v. Fructolysis Index
vi. Oxygen Utilization Test

15

Modern Semen Evaluation Techniques

Chetna Gangwar and Ravi Ranjan

Division of AP&R, ICAR-Central Institute for Research on Goats, Makhdoom Mathura- 281 122, Uttar Pradesh

Modern Semen Evaluation Methods

1. Fluorescent Microscopic Evaluation
2. In-vitro Fertility Test
3. Enzyme Estimation

1. Fluorescent Microscopic Evaluation

1.1. Acrosomal Integrity (Giemsa method and FITC-PSA assay)

The acrosomal integrity of the spermatozoa was detected using Fluorescence isothiocyanate – Pisum sativum agglutinin (FITC-PSA) staining procedure adopting method of Mendoza *et al.* (1992). Pisum sativum agglutinin (PSA) when conjugated to Lectin FITC marks the intact acrosome with bright green fluorescence. PSA is an agglutinin from edible pea that binds to glycoconjugates of acrosomal matrix or outer acrosomal membrane. It has affinity for terminal α –D-glucosyl and α-D-mannosyl residues of glycoproteins and it binds specifically to sugar α-mannoside found in acrosomal content.

Sperm suspension used for preparation of smear for FITC-PSA were washed (centrifugation with 1000 rpm for one minute) 2-3 times with DPBS (protein, calcium and magnesium free DPBS) solution as traces of protein on smear react with FITC labelled PSA and produces a strongly fluorescent background which makes the evaluation impossible. The smear prepared was air dried and dipped in absolute methanol for 30 seconds or 15 minutes and then allowed to dry rapidly. Methanol treated smears were then incubated for 30 minutes at room temperature in dark moisture chamber with FITC labelled PSA (50 μg/ml in DPBS). The slides were then washed in distilled water (rinsed with distilled water and further dipped in distilled water for 15 minutes) to remove unbound probe. The smear was air dried and examined immediately, without mounting, in an epifluorescence microscope.

Procedure

The entire procedure is described in a flow chart as under

Semen samples
(Fresh and post thaw)
↓
Washed (centrifugation @1000rpm for 1 min) with DPBS solution 3 x times
(Calcium, magnesium and protein free, pH 7.4 DPBS)
↓
Supernatant discarded
↓
Smear preparation, air dried and fixed with methanol for 15 min at room temperature
↓
Smear treated with FITC labeled PSA (50 µg/ml) in DPBS in a humified chamber at
room temperature for a minimum period of 30 minutes
↓
Slides rinsed in gentle stream of distilled water and dipped in distilled water for 15 minutes
↓
Smear air dried and observed under Fluorescence microsope (40X)

At least 200 spermatozoa must be counted in the prepared smear and differentiated according to the Fluorescence pattern of their acrosome as

S.No	Observation	Status of acrosome
01	Bright apple green fluorescence acrosome	Intact acrosome
02	No fluorescence or fluorescence at equatorial segment of acrosome	Damaged acrosome

1.1.1 Evaluation of capacitation status by Chlortetracycline assay (CTC Assay)

Capacitation status and acrosome reaction were assessed using Chlortetracycline (CTC) staining. The method used, was little modification of the earlier described method for goat (Fraser *et al.,* 1995). Chlortetracycline (CTC) binds with membrane calcium, whose distribution appears to change through capacitation, and is readily visualized by fluorescence microscopy. Hence, CTC distribution pattern seems to be related to the capacitation stage as well as status. Slides were observed using fluorescent under blue-violet illumination (excitation at 400–440 nm and emission at 470 nm by using 40× objective). A total of 200 sperm should be observed and different patterns of sperm were evaluated as established in literature. Three different forms of CTC pattern were observed namely,

a. **F pattern:** Even distribution of fluorescence over the entire head (uncapacitated sperm; pattern F).
b. **B pattern:** Fluorescence-free band in the post acrosomal region (capacitated, acrosome intact sperm; pattern B), fluorescence in anterior portion of the head.
c. **AR pattern:** Fluorescent free head except for a thin bright fluorescent band along the equatorial segment (acrosome-reacted cells, pattern AR).

Procedure

Sperm suspension (1×10^6/ml)

↓

Washing with TALP for 3 times (600×g) for 1 min

↓

Final pellet resuspended in 500 µl of TALP

↓

5mg of CTC stock was dissolved in 5ml of D.W

↓

500 µL of sperm suspension was added with 500µl of CTC Solution

↓

Incubation in dark for 30 min at 37^{0}C

↓

Washing of labeled cells at 500×g for 1 min (thrice)

↓

10 µl of cell suspension with cover slip

↓

Observation under fluorescence microscope by using UV filter

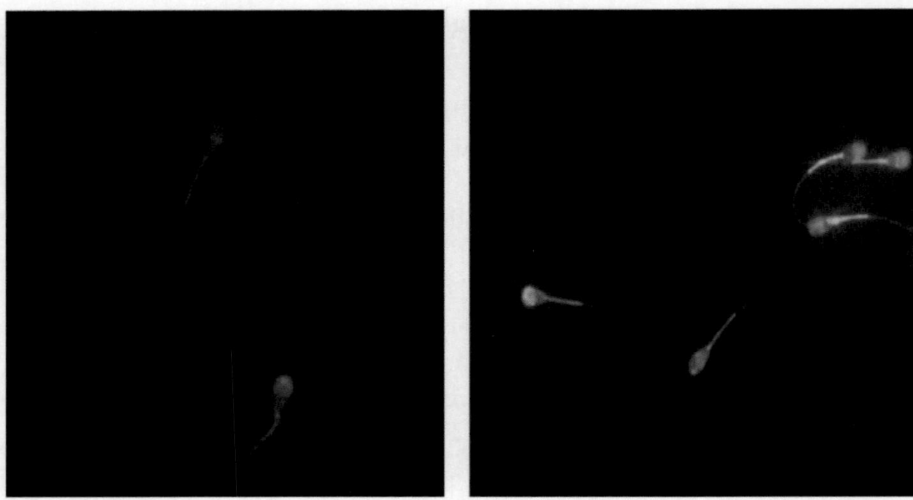

1.2. Evaluation of Mitochondria Transmembrane Potential

Mitochondria transmembrane potential was evaluated by using Mito Capture TM Apoptosis detection kit (Sigma, France). For mitochondrial transmembrane potential JC-1, assay was used. The method used was little modified from earlier described by Garner *et al.* (1994). The standard protocol specified in the kit was followed for the evaluation of the sperm. The kit employs a highly sensitive fluorochrome JC I for the detection of mitochondria transmembrane potential. With a higher inner transmembrane potential, JC I accumulates inside mitochondria and emits orange red fluorescence, whereas, a low transmembrane mitochondria potential causes JC I to get its monomer form and fluoresces green. Slides were observed using fluorescent microscope under blue-violet illumination (excitation at 400–440 nm and emission at 470 nm by using 40X objective). A total of 200 sperm per slide must be observed and different patterns of sperm were evaluated as per the site of fluorescence on the sperm.

Procedure

Sperm suspension (1×10^6/ml)

↓

Washing with for 3 times (600×g) for 1 min

↓

Final pellet resuspended in 500 μl of DPBS

↓

5mg of JC-1 stock was disolved in 5ml of DMSO

↓

500 μl of sperm suspension was added with 3 μl of JC-1

↓

Incubation in dark for 30 min at 37⁰C

↓

Washing of labeled cells at 500×g for 1 min (twice)

↓

10 μl of cell suspension with cover slip

↓

Observation under microscope by using blue filter

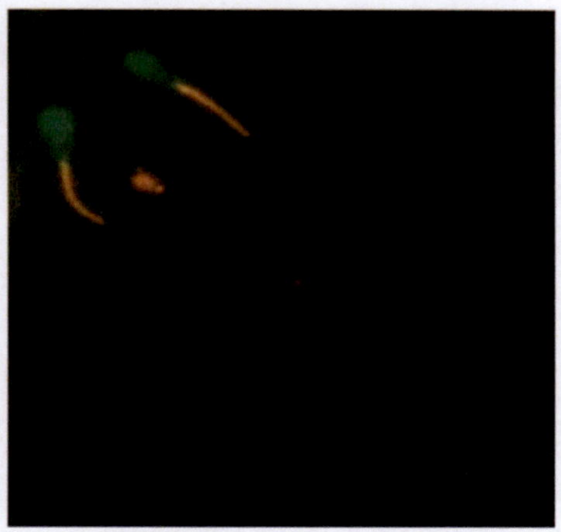

1.3. Evaluation of sperm apoptosis

Apoptotic cells undergo specific changes involving their structural and biochemical composition. Changes seen in sperm include; chromatin aggregation, cytoplasmic condensation, exposure of phosphatidyl serine (PS) on external on plasma membrane, DNA degradation and indentation of cytoplasmic and nuclear membrane. Annexin-V has biological property of binding phospholipids in a calcium dependent way. Annexin-V binds preferentially with phospholipids such as phosphatidyl serine which is normally not found in outer leaflet of plasma membrane. During early apoptosis plasma membrane phospholipids i.e., PS is translocated from inner to outer leaflet of lipid bilayer of plasma membrane thereby exposing PS to external cellular surface. Annexin-V has high affinity to bind with exposed PS which is a signal for early apoptosis.

S.No	Observation	Status of sperm
01	AN-/PI-	Live sperm
02	AN+/PI-	Apoptotic sperm
03	AN-/PI+	Dead sperm
04	AN+/PI+	Necrotic sperm

1.4. Evaluation of sperm DNA Damage

DNA damage can be assessed by

i) Sperm chromatin structure assay (SCSA)

ii) Terminal deoxynucleotidyl transferase dUTP nick end labeling (TUNEL Assay)

iii) Single cell gel Electrophoresis Assay (Comet Assay) etc.

Sperm chromatin structure assay (SCSA) is based on the assumption that structurally abnormal sperm chromatin is more susceptible to acid or heat denaturation. The sperm are thawed and a stress is applied by low pH. The DNA without single and double strand breaks is not susceptible to denaturizing conditions by pH=1.2. Disturbed chromatin integrity is characterized by presence of single and double strand breaks in DNA molecules that leads to formation of denatured single stranded segments (ss DNA). The SCSA method takes advantage of the metachromatic properties of acridine orange. The sperm are then labeled with a special dye called acridine orange. This dye fluoresces red when combine with the denatured DNA (ss DNA) while under some conditions with normal DNA (ss DNA) emits green fluorescence. A machine called a flow cytometer is used to analyze sperm from the sample. The sperm are passed in single file through a beam of light that hits the dye inside the sperm cell and reflects light at a specific wavelength causing the sperm to appear either orange (damaged) or green (normal). A computer counts the percentage of green versus orange-labelled sperm and software allows for creation of graphic plot of the percent of damaged sperm giving an index known as the DNA fragmentation index (DFI).

2. *In-vitro* Fertility Test

2.1 Cervical Mucus Penetration Test –

The semen deposited by natural service or Al has to be transported to the site of fertilization in the female genital tract. The sperm cells are transported through the cervical mucus, which is biochemically different from the seminal fluid. The cervical mucus penetration test gives a fairly good idea about the penetration capability of the spermatozoa through the cervical mucus. A highly significant positive correlation of ability of the spermatozoa to penetrate the cervical mucus and acrosome integrity and structural integrity of the spermatozoa has been reported. The limitation of this test lies on the fact that stage of estrum of the animal from which the mucus is collected. The storage time of the mucus also bears significant impact on the test results. Cervical mucus collected from animals which are not in proper stage of estrum and stored for prolonged period before being used the test may lead to erratic results.

Procedure

1. A Non heparinised capillary tube of 80 mm length and 0.8 mm diameter is taken.
2. One end of the capillary tube is sealed with PVA powder.
3. Place around 2 ml cervical mucus in a petri dish. Warm it to room temperature before use.
4. The cervical mucus is drawn in the capillary tube with the help of a scalp vein set attached to the capillary at one end (after removing the needle) and to a 5 ml syringe at the other end. The trailing mucus is then cut with scissors, leaving a small amount protruding from the filled end of the tube.
5. Remove the capillary tube from the loading manifold.
6. The open end of the capillary is then plugged with china clay.
7. The mucus filled capillary tubes are then allowed to stand at 37^0 C for 5 minutes.
8. Thaw a frozen semen straw and empty its contents into serum vial of 5ml capacity.
9. Suspend the capillary tube vertically into the serum vial and incubate it at 37 ° C for 30 minutes.
10. After 30 minutes of incubation, remove the capillary tube from the vial and wipe it with tissue paper to remove extra sperms adhering to the capillary tube.
11. Place the tube on a graduated microscope slide and observe the spermatozoa swimming in the mucus under 400 X magnification of the phase contrast microscope.

12. Measure the distance traveled by the spermatozoa in mm. This distance is called Sperm Penetration Distance (SPD). Semen sample with SPD 30 mm or more are considered to have better chance of fertilization.

2.2 Zona Binding Assay

The routine semen evaluation test needs to be combined with in vitro fertility tests to get a better prediction of sperm fertilization potential. Spermatozoa's close association with zona pellucida of ova can be used as vital characteristic exhibiting possible fertility of sperm. This association exhibits species specificity which is termed as attachment or zona binding.

Procedure

Sperm preparation

1. Two ml of frozen semen is taken and is diluted in 4 ml of mBWW medium.
2. The diluted semen is centrifuged for 15 min. at 300 g.
3. The supernatant is discarded and 2 ml of medium is added very slowly so that the sperm pellet is not disturbed.
4. Incubated at 37°C in air for one hour in slanting position for motile spermatozoa to swim up.
5. The supernatant is collected and centrifuged.
6. Discard the supernatant.

The sperm pellet is resuspended in MBWW to a final concentration of 10^6 ml spermatozoa per ml.

Prepration of Oocytes

1. Bovine ovaries are obtained from a slaughter house one day before the experiments and are kept in phosphate buffered saline (PBS) at 5^0C.
2. Antral follicle with a diameter of 4 to 8 mm are punctured and the aspirate of the follicular fluid is pooled in a petri dish.
3. Recover the cumulus oocytes complexes from the follicular fluid, collected in PBS and kept it for four minutes to remove cumulus cells. Mature oocytes have more cumulus mass.
4. The denuded oocytes are washed with PBS and kept at room temperature until they are incubated with spermatozoa.

Zona Binding Assay

1. Ten microliter droplet of 10^6 motile spermatozoa/ml are placed under mineral oil in 35 mm multi well petri dishes.
2. One or two oocytes are added to each droplet (at least 20 oocytes are used to estimate the sperm zona binding of each sample).
3. The gametes are incubated in CO_2 incubator for four hours.
4. After incubation, the oocytes –sperm complexes are rinsed five times with PBS, using a narrow-bore Pasteur pipette to remove loosely attached spermatozoa.
5. The sperm oocytes complexes are fixed with 2-5 % glutaraldehyde in 10 minutes washed with PBS, stained with 1 mg/ml Hoechst 33342 dye (Sigma) for 10 minutes and washed with PBS.
6. The Sperm oocytes complexes are placed on slide slightly compressed with a cover slip and sealed by paraffin/Vaseline.
7. The number of spermatozoa bound to the zona pellucid of the oocytes is counted under fluorescence microscope. If more than 200 sperms are attached, the sample is considered to have good fertility.

2.3 Hetero Spermic Insemination and Competitive Fertilization

This test is done to assess the relative fertilizing ability of the spermatozoon from two different bucks. The pooling of spermatozoa from two different buck is done prior to incubation with oocyte invitro. In this test identification of the source of each spermatozoon is essential. This may be achieved by the use of genetic markers or labeling of the spermatozoa.

2.4 Hemi-zona Assay

Hemizona assay is modification of the zona free hamster egg penetration test and heterospermic insemination and competitive fertilization. In this test spermatozoa from different bucks are incubated with hemi zona from a single oocyte. A significant relationship exists between the number of bound spermatozoa of a buck and the probability of pregnancy resulting from insemination with that buck's semen.

3. Enzyme Estimation

3.1 Hyaluronidase Activity

This enzyme is present in acrosomal system of spermatozoa. This enzyme has assumed a great importance in estimating fertilizing capacity of semen. If there is damage to the acrosome it is presumed that this enzyme will leak out in extracelluar fluid and presence of hyaluronidase activity in extracelluar fluid will indicate acrosomal damage. This is based on the estimation of N-acetylglucosamine liberated from hyaluronic acid by the enzyme. One unit the estimation of N-acetylglucosamine liberated from hyaluronic acid by the enzyme. One unit of hyaluronidase activity was defined as the amount of enzyme that cause the release of one micro mole of N- acetylglucosamine from hyaluronic acid at 37^0 C in 30 minutes. Release of hyaluronidase into extracellular fluid is an early and sensitive indication of damage sustained by acrosome. There is a significant release of enzyme into extracellular media due to freezing.

3.2 Alkaline/Acid Phosphatase Activity

Activity of alkaline phosphate in extracellular fluid is estimated by using P – nitrophenyl phosphate as substrate. Unit activity of enzyme is calculated as micro m of p-nitrophenol liberated per 100 ml in 30 minutes at 37°C. The alkaline and acid phosphates activity decreases significantly on freezing and storage in liquid nitrogen in all the diluents. The irreversible damage of enzyme proteins may be due to change in the three-dimensional configuration of the enzyme.

3.3 Acrosin Activity

Interest in acrosin developed when it was shown that the dispersion of zona pellucida from ova be sperm extract was due to proteinase. Acrosin, the main proteolytic enzyme in spermatozoa is used by the spermatozoa to penetrate the ovum's zona pellucida during fertilization. Three forms of acrosin have been detected in freshly collected semen. They are free acrosin, acrosin inhibitor complex and pro-acrosin. All three forms must be considered while analyzing total acrosin activity of spermatozoa. The enzyme activity is determined spectrophotometrically using alpha N- benzyl-L-arginine ethyl ester (BAEE) as a substrate. A significant decrease in the activity of the enzyme has been observed due to freezing of semen.

3.4 Lipid peroxidation by Malondialdehyde estimation

Lipid peroxidation level of spermatozoa was determined in frozen–thawed semen samples by measuring the MDA production, using thio-barbituric acid (TBA) as described by Kumaresan et al., (2006) with slight modifications in sperm concentration and incubation time. Frozen thawed semen (1 mL) mixed with 20% Trichloroacetic acid (TCA) and centrifuged at 960 g for 15 minutes. Then 1 mL supernatant was taken and mixed with 0.675% TBA and incubated at 95 C for 15 minutes. The absorbance was determined at 532 nm after cooling. The MDA concentration was determined by the specific absorbance coefficient (1.56×105 /molcm−3).

16

Buck Semen Cryopreservation

Chetna Gangwar, Ravi Ranjan and Manish Kumar

Division of AP&R, ICAR-Central Institute for Research on Goats, Makhdoom Mathura- 281 122, Uttar Pradesh

Introduction

Biological and chemical reactions in living cells are dramatically reduced at low temperature, a phenomenon that can lead to the possible long-term preservation of cells and tissues. However, freezing is fatal to most living organisms, since both intra and extracellular ice crystals are formed and results in changes to the chemical setting of cells that lead to cellular mechanical constraints and injury. The major hurdle for cells to overcome at low temperatures is the water-to-ice phase transition. Cell injury at fast cooling rates is attributed to intracellular ice formation, whereas slow cooling causes osmotic changes due to the effects of exposure to highly concentrated intra and extracellular solutions or to mechanical interactions between cells and the extracellular ice. Cryopreservation is a process that maintains biological samples in a state of suspended animation at cryogenic temperature for any considerable period and is used to preserve the fine structure of cells (Jang et al., 2017).

Advantages of semen cryopreservation

- Genetic improvement of livestock by higher utilization of outstanding male animals over an extended period.
- Disease control, in particular prevention of the transmission of infectious disease in the real ground for rational use of cryopreserved semen through A.I.
- A greater number of valuable males are at disposal to farmers at reasonable low cost.
- Cryopreserved semen can be transported easily throughout the world.

- Genetic progress is sooner provided for the evaluation of the genetic merit of the animal.
- Propagation of endangered animals can be possible through cryopreserved semen.

Disadvantages of semen cryopreservation

- Proper laboratory set up and skilled personals are required.
- Fertility through use of cryopreserved semen is low.

1. Types of semen preservation:

i) Preservation at room temperature (18-25^0 C)

ii) Preservation at refrigerator temperature (4-6^0 C)

iii) Preservation at ultra-low temperature (-79 to -196^0 C)

1.1 Semen preservation at room temperature

The diluter in which sperms are suspended at ambient temperature provide the condition which inhibits those pathways that are detrimental to their survival at higher temperature. CO_2 is very effective reversible inhibitor of sperm motility for short period, but prolonged exposure is toxic to sperm cells. On the basis of this principle, many extenders are designed which prevent sperm metabolism either by CO_2 gassing or producing CO_2 by chemical reaction. When CO_2 level is controlled properly, the motility and fertility of bull spermatozoa can be prolonged. CO_2 depresses motility and conserves energy of the cells. These extenders are not common because now a days we are using only frozen semen.

1.2 Semen preservation at refrigerator temperature

The refrigerator temperature lowers the metabolic rate of spermatozoa and in this way, it extends the fertile life of spermatozoa. Semen preserved at 5° C can be utilized for 2 to 4 days so that it is easy to be transported at distant locations. With refrigerated semen samples acceptable fertility using cervical insemination is obtained only up to 24 hours in sheep and 48 hours in goat.

1.3 Semen preservation at ultra low temperature

Cryopreservation or Semen preservation at ultra-low temperature refers to freezing and storage of semen at -79^0 C using dry ice and alcohol or at -196^0 C using liquid nitrogen gas as refrigerant. This can be achieved by either static vapour freezing (manual freezing method) or forced vapour freezing (freezing in a Programmable Bio- Freezer).

2. Principle of Cryopreservation

Cryopreservation includes several steps such as, dilution, cooling, freezing and thawing. The phenomena which cause damage to sperm cells during cryopreservation are mainly cold shock, solution effect and intracellular ice crystal formation. Cooling rate is vital factor determining the post thaw survival of the sperm cells. Cell death occurs in rapid freezing due to formation of intracellular and possibly extracellular ice. In contrast, slow cooling rates cause cell death due to diffusion of intracellular fluid into the extender, which then become increasingly hypertonic as the extender's water freezes causing intracellular osmotic damage as the cell dehydrates. Hence, the cooling rate needs to be balanced in a way that it is neither too fast to cause cell death due to cold shock nor too slow to result the same due to osmotic shock.

3. Methods of semen cryopreservation

- Manual Freezing Method
- Freezing in a Programmable Bio- Freezer

3.1 Manual Freezing Method

Horizontal liquid nitrogen vapour freezing technique is used for manual freezing of semen straws. This can be done in large liquid nitrogen storage containers or conventionally designed thermocool box. Semen straws are placed in liquid nitrogen vapours 4 cm above the level of liquid nitrogen for 10-15 minutes till they reach a temperature of -130^0 C to -150^{0}C and are then dipped into liquid nitrogen directly for further storage at -196^0 C.

3.2 Freezing in a Programmable Bio- Freezer

The equilibrated straws on a freezing rack are kept ready for loading. The liquid nitrogen container of the programmable freezer unit is filled with liquid nitrogen and the freezing unit is switched on and the already fed programme for freezing rate is selected. Run the programme and wait till the chamber temperature reaches 4^{0}C. At this stage the monitor will indicate "load samples". The samples loaded in the freezing chamber. The programme will run its course and when final temperature is reached, the monitor will indicate "remove samples" indicating that the freezing is completed. The straws are then collected in pre cooled goblets and immediately plunged into liquid nitrogen for further storage.

Cellular Damage Induced by Freezing

The process of cryopreservation exposes cells to stress induced by low-temperature and osmotic imbalances. Exposing biomolecules to decreasing temperatures may lead to (irreversible) conformational changes. Osmotic stress during cryopreservation is predominantly the result of extracellular ice formation. Upon extracellular ice formation, the solute concentration in the extracellular unfrozen fraction increases causing cells to dehydrate (Mazur, 2004; Meryman, 2007). Cellular dehydration during freezing is the result of water transport out of the cell in order to retain equilibrium between the intra and extracellular solute concentration. Dehydration especially occurs when low cooling rates are used. When cells shrink or swell beyond their osmotic tolerance limits this can be lethal (Benson et al., 2012). At fast cooling rates, cells do not have enough time to loosen water and as a result intracellular water contents remain relatively high leading to intracellular ice formation. Moreover, addition and removal of cryoprotective agents, also exposes cells to osmotic stress (Mazur, 2004; Kashuba et al., 2014; Meryman, 2007). Freezing also results in accumulation of damaging reactive oxygen species. Cryotolerance of spermatogonia stem cell is related to the extent ROS production in mitochondria. The 'two-factor hypothesis' postulates that cells display a specific optimal cooling rate, where damage due to dehydration (solute effects injury) and intracellular ice formation is minimal and cellular survival after thawing is maximal. The capacity of cells to change their volume in response to freezing-induced osmotic stress is determined by the rate of water transport into and out of the cells defined by the membrane hydraulic permeability and activation energy for water transport. The membrane permeability to water is determined by the membrane phospholipid composition, the presence of water and ion channel proteins, cytoskeletal elements (Elmoazzen et al., 2009), and is also altered by cryoprotective agents (Oldenhof et al., 2010). Cryoprotective agents increase membrane permeability to water, and thereby facilitate cellular dehydration during freezing even at low subzero temperatures (Xu et al., 2014). Moreover, cryoprotective agents typically shift the optimal cooling rate to lower temperatures and broaden the range of cooling rates resulting in optimal survival.

4. Different Types of Cryoprotective Agents

Cryopreservation requires protection of intracellular structures and biomolecules, and hence requires protective agents that are able to pass the cellular membrane.

a) Permeating cryoprotective agents are generally small non-ionic molecules. The most commonly used membrane permeable cryoprotective agents are dimethyl sulfoxide (DMSO) and glycerol. Alternatively, in cases where the above mentioned agents are toxic to the cells, ethylene glycol, methyl–formamide, or dimethyl–formamide may be used (Squires et al., 2004). Permeating cryoprotective agents are osmotically inactive, because they are equally distributed in the intracellular and extracellular spaces. However, addition itself poses osmotic stress to cells because water moves faster across the cellular membrane compared to the permeating cryoprotective agents. This result in an initial osmotic unbalance and shrinkage of the cells followed by an influx of water and cryoprotective agents until an equal distribution of cryoprotective agent inside and outside the cell is reached.

b) Non permeable cryoprotective agents can be divided into osmotically active molecules such as disaccharides (sucrose, trehalose) and osmotically inactive compounds including polysaccharides (hydroxyethyl starch, maltodextrin) and proteins (albumin, polyvinylpyrrolidone). Compounds such as sucrose are believed not to pass cellular membranes, and will cause cellular dehydration since they increase the osmolality of the cryopreservation medium. Addition of large macromolecules contributes little to the medium osmolality and this does not cause cellular dehydration. Protective effects of various proteins that are synthesized in response to stress have been investigated. Examples include antifreeze proteins, heat shock proteins (HSP), and so-called late embryo abundant (LEA) proteins.

Cryoprotective Agents (CPAs)

The CPA, reduces the freezing injury from the cryopreservation process. CPAs should be biologically acceptable and have low toxicity. Various CPAs have been developed and are used to reduce the amount of ice formed at any given temperature, depending on the cell type, cooling rate, and warming rate. In order to achieve the best survival rate of cells and tissues, the sample volume, cooling rate, warming rate, and CPA concentrations should be optimized depending on the different cell types and context of tissues. It should be mentioned that the macroscopic physical dimension of the tissue is a major point to be defined in a cryopreservation protocol because of heat and mass transfer limitations in these bulk systems. CPAs can be divided into two categories: (1) cell membrane permeating cryoprotectants, such as dimethyl sulfoxide (DMSO), glycerol and 1,2 propanediol; and (2) non-membrane-permeating cryoprotectants, such as 2-methy-2,4 pentanediol and polymers such as polyvinyl pyrrolidone, hydroxy ethyl starch, and various sugars. Unlike synthetic chemicals, biomaterials such as alginates, polyvinyl alcohol, and chitosan can be used to impede ice crystal growth, along with traditional small molecules. The direct inhibition of ice crystal formation and application of antioxidants and other compounds have been used to attempt to reduce cell death from processes such as apoptosis during the freezing and thawing cycle. Common CPAs are briefly addressed in the following subsections.

4.1 Glycerol

Polge et. al. discovered the cryoprotective effect of glycerol in 1949, and this polyol compound remained the most effective of additives until the protective effect of DMSO was demonstrated by Lovelock and Bishopin 1959. Glycerol is a nonelectrolyte and thus may act by reducing the electrolyte concentration in the residual unfrozen solution in and around a cell at any given temperature. It is widely used in the storage of animal sperm, bacteria and stem cells.

4.2 DMSO

First synthesized by the Russian scientist Alexander Zaytsevin 1866, DMSO has been commonly used for the cryopreservation of cultured mammalian cells because of its low cost and relatively low level of cytotoxicity. Like glycerol, DMSO acts by reducing the electrolyte concentration in the residual unfrozen solution in and around a cell at any given temperature. However, a decline in the survival rate and the induction of cell differentiation caused by DNA methylation and histone alteration has been reported.

4.3 Polymers

The entrapment of CPAs with in a capsule during cell resuspension in an encapsulating material is another strategy for the modulation of cell location. Among encapsulating materials, synthetic nonpenetrating polymers can provide cryoprotection (Best, 2015) of cells within the scaffold, there by bypassing the limitations of diffusion in higher dimensional cryopreservation. Vinyl-derived polymers, such as polyethylene glycol ($C_2nH_4n+2On+1$, molecular weight: 200–9500Da), polyvinyl alcohol [(C_2H_4O) n, molecular weight: 30–70kDa], and hydroxyethyl starch (130–200 kDa), have a capacity to decrease the size of formed ice crystals.

4.4 Sugars

Sugars have cryoprotective properties and are not toxic, hence trehalose has been investigated as an alternative CPA by virtue of its stability upon freezing. Trehalose is a disaccharide found at high concentration in a variety of organisms capable of surviving in complete dehydration, including bacteria, yeast and nematodes. Mammals do not produce trehalose but indeed it is an effective cryoprotectant, decreasing the amount of cell injury by ice crystallization (Ntai et al., 2018). Its protective action is related both to osmotic effect and specific interactions with cell membrane phospholipids and labile proteins, preventing their damage and denaturation due to desiccation and oxidative stress (Benaroudj et al., 2001). Nevertheless, the precise mechanism by which trehalose provides such protection is yet to be elucidated.

4.5 Proteins

Sericin is a water-soluble sticky protein (~30 kDa) isolated from the silkworm cocoon and has been developed as a fetal bovine serum or DMSO replacing CPA for Semen cryopreservation, or hepatocytes (Reddy et al., 2018). Small antifreeze proteins derived from marine teleost or fishes have also attracted attention as CPAs.

5. Limitations of cryopreservation

Although numerous usages of the cryopreservation technique exist, both in basic and clinical research, some limitations still exist. Cells metabolize almost nothing at low temperatures such as $-196^{0}C$ (i.e., in liquid nitrogen), which has inevitable side effects, including a genetic drift toward biological variations of cell-associated changes in lipids and proteins that could result in the impairment of cellular activity and structure. If there were no limit to the amount of CPA that could be used, cells would be preserved perfectly. In conventional settings, however, CPAs themselves can be damaging to cells, especially when used in high concentrations. For example, there is a possibility that DMSO may alter chromosome stability, which can lead to a risk of tumor formation. Apart from endogenous changes in cells, the possible infection or contamination with cells such as tumorous ones should be prevented.

References

Benaroudj N, Lee DH, Goldberg AL (2001). Trehalose accumulation during cellularstress protects cells and cellular proteins from damage by oxygen radicals. The J. Biol.Chem. 276 (26), 24261–24267.

Benson JD, Woods EJ, Walters EM, Critser JK (2012). The cryobiology of spermatozoa. Theriogenology 78, 1682–1699.

Best BP (2015). Cryoprotectant toxicity: facts, issues, and questions. Rejuvenation Res 18:422–36.

Elmoazzen HY, Elliott JA, McGann LE (2009). Osmotic transport across cell membranes in nondilute solutions: a new nondilute solute transport equation. Biophys. J. 96, 2559- 2571.

Holm F, Ström S, Inzunza J, Baker D, Strömberg AM, Rozell B (2010). An effective serum- and xeno-free chemically definedfreezing procedure for human embryonic and inducedpluripotent stem cells. Hum Reprod 25, 1271–9.

Jang T H, Park S C, Yang J H, Kim J Y, Seok J H, Park U S, Choi C W, Leeb S R, Han J (2017). Cryopreservation and its clinical applications. Integr Med Res 6, 12–18.

Kashuba, CM, Benson JD, Critser JK (2014). Rationally optimized cryopreservation of multiple mouse embryonic stem cell lines: I--Comparative fundamental cryobiology of multiple mouse embryonic stem cell lines and the implications for embryonic stem cell cryopreservation protocols. Cryobiology 68, 166–175.

Li Y, Tan JC, Li LS (2010). Comparison of three methods forcryopreservation of human embryonic stem cells. Fertil Steril 93, 999–1005.

Mazur P (2004). Principles of cryobiology.in Fuller, B.J., Lane, N.L., Benson, E.E. (Eds.), Life in the frozen state. CRC Press LLC, Boca Raton, FL, pp 3–65.

Meryman HT (2007). Cryopreservation of living cells: principles and practice. Transfusion.47, 935–945.

Ntai A, Spada A L, Blasio P D, Biunno I (2018). Trehalose to cryopreserve human pluripotent stem cells. Stem Cell Research 31, 102–112.

Oldenhof H, Friedel K, Sieme H, Glasmacher B, Wolkers WF (2010). Membrane permeability parameters for freezing of stallion sperm as determined by Fourier transform infrared spectroscopy. Cryobiology 61, 115–122.

Reddy VS, Yadav B, Yadav CL, Anand M, Swain DK, Kumar D, Kritania D, Madan AK, Kumar J, Yadav S. Effect of sericin supplementation on heat shock protein 70 (HSP70) expression, redox status and post thaw semen quality in goat. Cryobiology 84, 33-39.

Xu Y, Zhao G, Zhou X, Ding W, Shu Z, Gao, D (2014). Biotransport and intracellular ice formation phenomena in freezing human embryonic kidney cells (HEK293T). Cryobiology 68, 294–302.

17

Advances in Buck Semen Cryopreservation Insight into Semen Extenders

[1]Prabhat Kumar Pankaj, [2]Chetna Gangwar and [2]R. Pourouchottamane

[1]Division of Transfer of Technology, ICAR- Central Research Institute for Dryland Agriculture, Santoshnagar- 500 059, Hyderabaad
[2]Division of AP&R, ICAR-Central Institute for Research on Goats Makhdoom, Mathura- 281 122, Uttar Pradesh

All living organisms need to reproduce in order to maintain their species and improve the economics of animal husbandry. Since the beginning of time, different methods of successful reproduction have been created, including artificial insemination and *in vitro* fertilization. To shield sperm from damaging elements like freezing, osmotic shock, oxidative stress, and cell damage by ice crystals, semen extenders were developed. Semen extenders maintain sperm's characteristics, such as its morphology, motility, and viability as well as its membrane, acrosomal, and DNA integrity. To improve semen quality for fertilization, semen extenders must offer a suitable pH, adenosine triphosphate, anti-cooling and anti-freeze shock, and antioxidant activity. As a result, this compilation of research offers exact information on various semen extenders, preservation mechanisms, and crucial semen extender additions in goats. By incorporating various types of additives in semen extenders for cryopreservation, significant improvement is reported in post thaw sperm quality in terms of increased % motility, viability, PMAI, MMP and reduced DNA fragmentation, capacitation like changes reflected by less CTC pattern B and AR, Tyrosine Phosphorylated pattern A, E and AE.

Artificial insemination (AI) is a potent and one-of-a-kind method forfertilizing the females of most mammals. AI was supposed to improve the number of insemination dosages from a single ejaculate but failed due to the lack of sperm-washing techniques for both chilled and frozen-thawed male donor sperm in goats. AI can have an impact on many productivity projects of goat husbandry and boosting weaning weight, to improve economic efficiency. As a result, AI has a remarkable potential to influence economic feasibility. Furthermore, AI requires fresh or well-preserved sperm, and overall 95% of the preserved sperm is used in all AI. To maintain its quality, sperm must be stored in a suitable medium. As a result, semen extenders used to maintain semen during chilling or cryopreservation must be developed and evaluated. This review contains detailed information on semen extenders, semen preservation processes, and necessary additions for goat semen extenders.

Buck sperm varies from stallion and boar sperm in that it is composed of a modest volume (a few mL) of seminal plasma with a high concentration of spermatozoa. Globally, reproductive research in livestock has tended to focus on cattle and pigs rather than small ruminants, resulting in less advanced sperm handling and cryopreservation for AI in the latter. Furthermore, the structure of the female reproductive canal in these animals is more difficult to navigate than in cattle, as the cervix is firmly curled, making insertion of the insemination catheter problematic. Productivity in goats could be boosted by enhancing the quality of spermatozoa used in AI and the AI techniques used in these species.

AI in goats has typically been conducted using fresh or cooled spermatozoa, with satisfactory reproductive results. However, the use of foreign breeds, genetic enhancement, and the use of safe semen from other nations necessitates the use of frozen semen in order to complete analyses for pollutants or diseases in the donor male before the semen doses are used for AI. Although the post-thaw motility of frozen sperm from goats is generally deemed acceptable, low fertility has been associated with its usage in AI, owing to the spermatozoa's reduced lifespan.

In goats, the sperm cryopreservation process is a challenge, requiring improvements that maximize the viability and fertility of the gametes after thawing. To date, very less significant results have been obtained with AI, using frozen semen of this species. Contributing to this situation, goat breeders present the enzyme phospholipase A in their seminal plasma, which is secreted by the bulbourethral glands, and interacts with the phospholipids and triglycerides, present in seminal extenders based on milk or egg yolk. From the lecithin and triglyceride hydrolysis, catalyzed by phospholipase A, harmful components to sperm are generated, which are represented by lysolecithin and toxic fatty acids, respectively. As a result, for goat semen cryopreservation in milk and egg yolk extenders it is necessary to remove the seminal plasma, by centrifugation, before semen dilution is performed. However, it is known that centrifugation can damage the gametes, increasing the production of reactive oxygen species (ROS) and the oxidative stress

The complex anatomy of the doe's cervix is a major factor affecting the pregnancy rate obtained with frozen-thawed buck semen. In the cervical canal, the anatomical structure of several rings limits the passing of the insemination pipette towards the uterus for AI. These rings provide a physical barrier to external contamination but also present a major barrier to transcervical AI. Fertility following AI with cryopreserved semen is also limited by the inability of frozen-thawed spermatozoa to transit the cervix. Data indicate that, in order to achieve high pregnancy rate with cryopreserved spermatozoa, semen must be deposited directly into the uterine lumen, next to the oviduct, close to the site of ovulation either with a laparoscopic intrauterine insemination technique or a trans-cervical intrauterine procedure. Also, the preservation of buck semen, whether cooled or cryopreserved, is difficult because of toxic interactions between seminal plasma and milk/egg-yolk-based extenders. Insemination of does with fresh semen yields fertilization rates comparable to those obtained by natural mating. In both ewes and does, transcervical AI would be even simpler if it were sufficient to deposit the semen in only one uterine horn. Generally, the timing of AI depends on the AI method used, the nature of oestrus (spontaneous or induced), the type of semen (fresh diluted/undiluted or frozen), the age and breed of the animal, and whether single or double AI is to be performed.

Preservation of Semen

Except for the removal of seminal plasma, the goat semen freezing technique adheres to basic principles shared by other species. The sperm should be diluted in a suitable medium that provides a favourable environment for its longevity and fertility. As a result, the seminal extender should act as a buffer, nutritional supplement, and cryoprotectant. This is due to osmotic alterations, pH oscillations, energy depletion during metabolism, thermal shock and cryodamage, changes in membrane composition, and ROS formation, all of which cause injuries to the gametes during cryopreservation. Chilling and cryopreservation are the two main methods for storing sperm. For the chilling process, semen is kept at 4-5°C for three days to achieve the optimum results. Semen is frozen for 3 hours at 4°C in the cryopreservation procedure. Meanwhile, it is put into 0.25-ml straws and then preserved and stored for years in liquid nitrogen. As a result, the most important components for long- term semen preservation include cooling for 2-3 hours, adding a cryoprotectant, and freezing in liquid nitrogen.

Cooling Temperature for Semen Preservation

During liquid storage, the temperature is reduced to promote sperm inactivity. To maintain semen quality and minimize gamete metabolism in goats, the cooling temperature should be kept between 4°C and 5°C, whereas in boars, the diluted liquid semen should be held between 15°C and 17°C. Rapid temperature drops harm mammalian sperm cells. The temperature of post-chilled sperm may not be as damaging to male sperm integrity as the post-thawed approach, which results in low spermatozoa value. A significant advantage of utilizing cooled semen is the higher fertility % as compared to freeze-thawed semen, which reduces the insemination dose and increases the dose number, lowering storage costs and simplifying the usage of AI. Furthermore, cooled sperm has a longer lifespan in the female reproductive system than frozen sperm and a higher conception rate.

Cryopreservation of Semen

Cryopreservation is the freezing of sperm, a process used to preserve cells and tissues alive in liquid nitrogen at -196°C. The modern cryobiology era saw the introduction of liquid nitrogen. Other advantages of cryopreservation include long-distance transportation of precious genetic resources and the prevention of disease spread. A single dose of cryopreserved sperm can accomplish 8 times more *in vivo* fertilization than fresh sperm. However, because of the exposure to ambient oxygen, semen cryopreservation creates free radicals and eliminates seminal plasma from the sperm cells. This causes sperm cells to produce lipid peroxidation, which promotes the creation of reactive oxygen species (ROS). The advancement of cryopreservation techniques and sperm extenders has considerably reduced the negative effects of cryopreservation.

The issue during cryopreservation is not the ability of sperm cells to withstand the liquid nitrogen storage time, but rather navigating the intermediate temperature zone. These temperatures must be passed through the cells twice, once during cooling and once during thawing, causing harm to the integrity of the sperm plasma membrane, acrosome, and nucleus, as well as mitochondrial function and sperm motility. Conventional freezing, directed freezing, and sperm vitrification are all cryopreservation procedures. Dimethyl sulfoxide (DMSO) and propylene glycol (PG) are two anti-freezing cryoprotectants. For best results, maintain a cryoprotectant concentration of 5-15% during freezing and thawing of isolated cells.

Development of semen extender

Experts have created material to help sperm survive cooling and freezing processes. Many obstacles were confronted and overcome, including media toxicity, variable pH, ROS, energy source, sperm membrane damage, and cryo-shock preservatives. Extenders protect sperm, maintain motility and fertility over time by stabilizing the plasmalemma, provide energy substrates, and guard against the negative effects of pH and osmolarity fluctuations. These techniques make it possible to boost the rate of fertilization by utilizing high-quality extenders during chilling and cryopreservation. As a result, higher-quality sperm extenders and additions should be used to improve sperm quality and raise the rate of sperm fertilization.

Semen extender

Semen extenders are used to preserve sperm in order to facilitate conception. Semen extenders can also keep sperm metabolic processes going, manage the pH of the medium during and after post-thawing, prevent bacterial transmission and contamination, and limit cryogenic damage. Similarly, semen extenders must have other properties such as keeping the pH between 6.8 and 7.2, providing energy, antioxidants to reduce oxidative stress, antibiotics to avoid contamination, and anti-freezing shock. These qualities preserve sperm preservation and transit, allowing it to be employed in AI IVF, intra-cytoplasmic sperm injection, and research studies. Extenders come in two varieties: chilled (liquid form) for 3 days on average and cryopreserved for years. Currently, multiple extenders use various material sources such as animal source, egg yolk, skimmed milk, and plant source (soybean lecithin), which acts as an emulsifier, or lubricant and other varied features depending on the type of sperm extender and species. The fact that soybean-lecithin based semen extender is more hygienic than egg yolk extender is a plus. Because of their low cost and good outcomes, egg yolk semen extenders are widely utilized in laboratory and field approaches.

Various Components of Semen Extender Non-penetrating cryoprotectant source

Skim milk and egg yolk are widely used as non-penetrating cryoprotectants for preserving sperm of different male mammals. Because these extenders might protect sperm membranes, their acrosome and DNA may be damaged because of high lecithin content. Furthermore, soybean-lecithin extenders can substitute the animal source as a source of lipid/lipoprotein.

Egg Yolk: Egg yolk is the primary non-penetrate substance used in extenders to dilute semen and protect sperm from freeze shock during the chilling process. Egg yolk-based extender is commonly used in chilled, frozen semen, or both. It works as a reservoir of cholesterol and phospholipids that help protect the sperm cell membrane and acrosome against cryogenic injury. Furthermore, it prevents the loss of membrane phospholipids during the freezing process. Egg yolk protein has hydrophobic properties, which cannot penetrate the cell wall of sperm. The low-density lipoprotein (LDL) of egg yolk maintains sperm membrane phospholipids throughout the cryopreservation processes. The previous works have shown that sperm are protected during freezing by sequestering lipid-binding proteins from LDL in the egg yolk. It is also considered a source of long-chain polyunsaturated fatty acids. Besides, egg yolk contains lipid, protein and carbohydrate; it also contains minerals.

In contrast, several drawbacks against egg yolk-based semen extender use include the wide range of variability in the composition of egg yolk, the risk of disease transmission or bacterial contamination, and involvement of egg yolk in the microscopic examination of semen. In general, egg yolk is used in semen extenders at different concentrations. However, it was also used at 20% (v/v). Studies revealed that LDLs are the egg yolk active ingredients responsible for sperm protection.

Two types of extenders can be prepared from egg yolk:

Egg yolk-based extender: Here, the concentration of the egg yolk is 20%. Tris-buffered egg yolk extenders containing fructose and glycerol preserve the fertility of animal sperm at high extension rates.

LDL extender: LDL (w/v) was prepared in the laboratory by ultracentrifugation. Higher kinetic parameters were achieved using 2%, 4%, and 8% LDL compared with 20% whole egg yolk in a Tris-milk extender and can lower the concentration of LDL, such as 2% associated with skimmed milk, which can be used for buffalo semen freezing. According to several studies, egg yolk can be used with a 20% extender concentration. In contrast, LDL can be used with 8% concentration, and 2% LDL can be added solely with skimmed milk. One significant challenge of using egg yolk and its derivatives is microbial contamination by *Escherichia coli*. Consequently, the fertilization capacity of contaminated semen could negatively affect the risk of microbial contamination associated with the egg yolk extender.

Milk Sources: Milk has been adapted for freezing mammalian semen mostly in a reconstituted form combined with arabinose, fructose, or egg yolk. Skim milk proteins buffer semen pH and may also chelate any heavy metal ions. An important milk compound is lactose, which is hydrophilic and cannot diffuse the cell wall of the sperm cells, which protects the cell wall and prevents freeze shock. Skim milk-based extender is superior to TRIS-based extender based on semen preservation.

Soybean Lecithin: Soybean lecithin is an alternative for egg yolk and has been developed and used commercially for semen preservation. Lecithin from soybean has been successfully used for semen cryopreservation. Nowadays, researchers believe that extenders free from animal ingredients can decrease the risk of contamination transported by the animal source. Therefore, soybean lecithin can be used as an alternative to milkor egg yolk-based extenders for semen cryopreservation in bulls, rams and bucks. The active components of soybean lecithin and egg yolk are entirely identical. These components are oleic acid, palmitic acid, stearic acid, and phosphatidylcholine. They prevent the diluted semen from freeze shock. The prevailing phospholipids in most mammalian biological membranes can confer physical stability to sperm cells. Semen extender supplemented with soybean lecithin at 6% could upgrade sperm general and progressive motility and intact plasma membrane of post-thawed male boar sperm cells. Tris-soybean lecithin-based extender at a 3% concentration can be an appropriate alternative to either BullXcell® or OptiXcell® in Damascus goat sperm cryopreservation.

Glycerol as an anti-shock: After discovering glycerol as a remarkable cryoprotective agent for cryopreserving semen, using liquid nitrogen for adequate storage of frozen semen and AI has been a valuable and prevalent reproductive biotechnology for cattle genetic improvement. Discovering the cryoprotective properties of glycerol in 1949 enabled the cryopreservation of different animals' sperm. Although different cryoprotective substances have been tested, including dimethyl sulphoxide (DMSO) and propanediol (PROH), glycerol remains the favorite cryoprotectant for semen cryopreservation. Glycerol is a dominant cryoprotectant that can cross the cell membrane. Studies stated that glycerol could be added to the semen at different temperatures. Semen extenders containing egg yolk with 6% glycerol, followed by a rapid cooling rate, could yield higher post-thaw outcomes for epididymal sperm compared with semen extenders containing 3% glycerol. DMSO is a cryoprotectant that quickly enters sperm cells. It can be used to maintain the frozen sperm quality of bulls, boars, goats, and dogs. Ethylene glycol is more dominantly used in buffalos, bulls, and sheep.

Source of Energy: Energy intake is responsible for the continuation of development and the function of all living cells, and gametes are no exception. Two metabolic pathways are producing adenosine triphosphate (ATP), that supplies energy for the main functions of sperm, which are oxidative phosphorylation and glycolysis. Glycolysis occurs in the cytoplasm of sperm cells and provides energy for sperm metabolism. Sugar, such as fructose and glucose, is considered the primary energy source in sperm cells. However, fructose is the best sugar for maintaining functional membrane integrity, adequate sperm motility, and tonic after thawing.

Disaccharides are considered non-permeating agents for cells. These sugars interact with phospholipids of the plasma membrane, increasing sperm survival post-cryopreservation. Moreover, lactate and pyruvate are significant energy sources in stallion sperm with dose effects on mitochondrial function, motility, and ROS production. Trehalose can be used as a cryoprotectant in semen extenders to preserve the optimal quality of motility, viability, and membrane integrity of goat sperm cells compared with other types of sugar. Glucose is a component of egg yolk and, therefore, can be used as an energy source. Nonetheless, other kinds of sugars, such as galactose, sucrose, maltose, xylose, and raffinose, have been successfully used for frozen bull semen.

Various Components as Additives to Semen Extenders

To promote the quality of the extenders, several studies have been undertaken to use different materials and compounds such as those of plant origins, whole milk, fish oil, and honey, which contain natural compounds such as antioxidants. A compilation of such additives with different semen extenders are displayed in Table 1.

Table 1. Major Additives used during semen extension for chilled and frozen semen storage*

Additives	Extenders	Mechanism of action	Effect
Cysteine (0.2%) (Buffalo semen) (4-7 ^{0}C) (96 hrs)	Citric-whey extender	-SH group of cysteine destroy lactenin (spermicidal toxin)	Increase motility (45%) and non-eosinophilic spermatozoa (51%)
Iodixanol (2.5 %) (Cattle semen)	Tris-egg yolk	Non-penetrating cryoprotectant (altering ice crystal formation at lower temperatures)	Increase progressive motility (27.33%), viability (85.33%), Plasma membrane acrosomal integrity (PMAI) (59.94%)
Soy-lecithin (25%) (Bovine semen) (5 ^{0}C) (72hr)	Soya milk based-extender	Lecithin protects plasma membrane by restoring phospholipids	Enhances sperm membrane (48.3%) and acrosome integrity (93.3%), viability (48.3%) & motility (43.9%)

Coconut water (Buffalo semen)	CEBRAN-I diluter	Indole-3-acetic acid (IAA) – inhibits enzyme phospholipase-2 (PLA2)	Increase motility (38.8%), viability (61%) and less acrosomal damage (10.4%)
Regucalcin (40 µg/ml) (Buffalo semen)	Tris-citric acid-fructose-egg yolk-glycerol	Ca^{2+} homeostasis and antioxidant property, stimulate gluconolactonase enzyme	Increase in post-thaw progressive motility (50.6%), acrosome integrity (75.6%) and ZP binding (191.9)
Curcumin (diferuloylmethane) (1.5 mM) (Buffalo semen)	Tris-citric acid extender	Radical trapping-antioxidant (H-atom transfer from CH2 group atthe centre of the heptadione link along with that of its phenolic –OH group	High progressive motility (23.27%), rapid velocity (31.53%) and other secondary motion characteristics, high plasma membrane integrity (30.47%) and viable spermatozoa with intact acrosome (61.87%)
Astaxanthin (2µM) (Karan Fries semen) (5°C)(72 hrs)	Tris-egg yolk-citric acid fructose	Antioxidant property	Increase progressive motility (72.5%), % of live sperm (80.92%) and reduce levels of catalase (14.43U/ml) and SOD (30 U/ml)
Soy lecithin (1.5 %) with 2% virgin coconut oil (VCO)(4 °C) (72hr)	Tris-based extender (egg yolk free)	VCO contains antioxidants such as tocotrienol, polyphenols, and tocopherols	improves sperm viability (64.83%), acrosome integrity (75.5%), morphology (97.96%), membrane integrity (62.29%) and lipid peroxidation status-MDA (23 nmol/sample)
Diospyros kaki (Cattle semen) (for chilled and frozen semen)	Tris-Citrate-Fructose egg yolk	Antioxidant property(due to high level of carotenoids, flavonoids and polyphenols)	Increase post-thaw sperm motility (57%), higher conception rate (67%)

Lycopene (1.5 mmol/l) (natural carotenoid) (Bovine semen)	Triladyl®	Scavenger of singlet oxygen ($^1O2$) and other ROS	High progressive motility (43.01%) and improved secondary motion characteristics, plasma membrane stability (84.90%), acrosomal Integrity (85.20%), mitochondrial activity (147.50%), low intracellular superoxide generation (42.58%) and MDA (2.43 μmol/gprotein)
Regucalcin (40 μg/ml) (Buffalo semen)	Tris-citric acid-fructose-egg yolk-glycerol	Ca^{2+} homeostasis and antioxidant property, stimulate gluconolactonase enzyme	Increase in post-thaw progressive motility (50.6%), acrosome integrity (75.6%) and ZP binding (191.9)
Curcumin (diferuloylmethane) (1.5 mM) (Buffalo semen)	Tris-citric acid extender	Radical trapping-antioxidant (H-atom transfer from CH2 group atthe centre of the heptadione link along with that of its phenolic –OH group	High progressive motility (23.27%), rapid velocity (31.53%) and other secondary motion characteristics, high plasma membrane integrity (30.47%) and viable spermatozoa with intact acrosome (61.87%)
Astaxanthin (2μM) (Karan Fries semen) (5^0C)(72 hrs)	Tris-egg yolk-citric acid fructose	Antioxidant property	Increase progressive motility (72.5%), % of live sperm (80.92%) and reduce levels of catalase (14.43U/ml) and SOD (30 U/ml)
Soy lecithin (1.5 %) with 2% virgin coconut oil (VCO)(4 °C) (72hr)	Tris-based extender (egg yolk free)	VCO contains antioxidants such as tocotrienol, polyphenols, and tocopherols	improves sperm viability (64.83%), acrosome integrity (75.5%), morphology (97.96%), membrane integrity (62.29%) and lipid peroxidation status-MDA (23 nmol/sample)

Diospyros kaki (Cattle semen) (for chilled and frozen semen)	Tris-Citrate-Fructose egg yolk	Antioxidant property(due to high level of carotenoids, flavonoids and polyphenols)	Increase post-thaw sperm motility (57%), higher conception rate (67%)
Lycopene (1.5 mmol/l) (natural carotenoid) (Bovine semen)	Triladyl®	Scavenger of singlet oxygen ($^{1}O2$) and other ROS	High progressive motility (43.01%) and improved secondary motion characteristics, plasma membrane stability (84.90%), acrosomal Integrity (85.20%), mitochondrial activity (147.50%), low intracellular superoxide generation (42.58%) and MDA (2.43 μmol/gprotein)
Coenzyme Q10 (ubiquinone) (30 μM) (Bovine semen)	Tris-egg yolk	Prevents LPO and DNA fragmentation (lipid soluble antioxidant and scavenge free radicals)	Increase post thaw motility (65.8%), livability (68.3%), plasma membrane (67.9%) and acrosome integrity (22.9% damage acrosome), lowers sperm abnormalities (22.7%) with reduced levels of AST (25.1 IU/l) and ALT (21.7 IU/l)
Melatonin (2.0 and 3.0 mM) (Bovine semen)	Citrate- egg yolk	Sequester and neutralize free radicals, electron donation, stimulate glutathione peroxidase (GSH-Px), catalase, and SOD	Increase post thaw sperm motility (30.1%), viability (69.8%),plasma membrane integrity (68.3%), normal sperm (93.1%), and antioxidant enzymes activity)

*Adopted from Nitin *et al.*, 2018.

Added Components of Plant Origin: There is an international demand for using natural medical sources in semen extenders of different animals, for example, strawberry, green tea, virgin coconut oil, pomegranate, and *Pinus brutia*, among others. The effects of several plant extracts on fertility have been demonstrated as antioxidants in many animal species due to their free radical scavenging properties. Researchers found that supplementation of Tris-citric acid extender with 1.0% green tea improved sperm parameters in both *in vitro* and *in vivo* fertilization, which decreased lipid peroxidation in buffalo bull sperm freezing and thawing processes. For virgin oil addition, researchers found that Tris-based extenders containing 2% virgin oil did not improve the quality of parameters for freeze–thawed bull semen but enhanced the quality of parameters for chilled bull semen. An experimental study illustrated that adding *P. brutia* to the semen extender does not improve parameters such as motility but prevents chromatin damage and reduces oxidative stress and sperm abnormalities when used at a concentration of 50 mg/ml.

Added components of animal origin

Honey: Adding honey to extenders significantly affected sperm motility before freezing and sperm abnormality of the freeze–thawed semen. Honey contains a high number of various simple sugars and antioxidants. Furthermore, honey is also a highly concentrated product. It has a potential hyperosmotic extracellular environment around sperm cells that enhance the efflux of intracellular fluid, thereby minimizing the formation of ice crystals inside the sperm cytoplasm, which has been linked to sperm damage during cryopreservation. This illustrated that using honey increased the quality of the semen after thawing compared with using egg yolk extenders.

In addition, researchers have reported the benefits of using honey as a supplement in the cryopreservation semen media of various animals, such as goat, which act as natural antibiotics against pathogenic bacteria, hinder sperm survival, fertilizing ability, reduce the number of dead abnormal sperm, and acrosomal damage. Some studies showed that using 2.5% honey might be an energy source to ram semen.

Fish oil: Fish oil can improve semen performance after freeze–thawing and AI besides the type of extender shown in bulls. The addition of 150 mg/100 mL fish oil in the extender could positively enhance the quality of post-thawed semen. Adding 0.30 g of fish oil per 100 ml of egg yolk-based extender resulted in an improved fertility capacity of ram and goat semen. Some studies reported that the addition of fish oil to feed supplements improved the semen quality and fertility rate of sheep and goat.

Vitamins: Vitamins are added to extenders to improve semen function parameters for liquid nitrogen storage or cryopreserved sperm cells because vitamins are non-enzymatic antioxidants.

Vitamin B12: Adding Vitamin B12 to the extenders improved bull frozen semen quality, elevated the motility percentage of sperm cells, and improved movement characteristics. Researchers found that the addition of 2.50 mg/ml Vitamin B_{12} to semen extenders improved bull frozen semen parameters and quality.

Vitamin E: Vitamin E is a cellular stabilizer of unsaturated lipids against oxidative deterioration, and hence, it maintains the structural and functional integrity at the subcellular level. In general, Vitamin E is the primary component of the antioxidant system in sperm cells. Furthermore, adding Vitamin E to Tris-egg yolk extenders at 60 and 120 μM provides higher integrity to the plasma membrane, mitochondria, and kinematic parameters of sperm cells of rams and bucks post-cryopreservation.

Vitamin C: Vitamin C is the most crucial antioxidant in seminal fluid. Researchers found that 0.9 mg/mL of Vitamin C improves the longevity and quality of chilled sperm in Awassi ram semen stored at 5^0C. Furthermore, as an alternative to glutathione, Vitamin C is considered more efficient in protecting ram sperm viability and acrosomal integrity than Vitamin E because Vitamin C can neutralize H_2O_2 production in a hydrophilic environment by preventing peroxide formation. However, higher concentrations of Vitamin C (2.5 mM) proved to be harmful to sperm motility in freeze-thawed bull semen.

Other Additions

Several researchers have added various substances to semen extenders, such as milk, caseinate, and lactoferrin. Other researchers added hormones, such as insulin, follicle-stimulating hormone, and testosterone, to the semen extenders. The addition of selenium improved male reproductive performance by potentiating semen quality and suppressing free radicals. Selenium could decrease lipid peroxidation and increase antioxidants in rooster seminal plasma after the freeze–thawing process.

Antibiotic addition to semen extenders: Antibiotic is added to semen extenders to reduce microbial contamination of the external environment or during semen collection. Different antibiotics, such as penicillin and streptomycin, ceftiofur, apramycin, and aminoglycosides or linco-spectin + tylosin + gentamycin, have been added to semen extenders.

Commercial extenders

Several commercial extenders are used for diluting and preserving semen during cooling and cryoprotection. Optidyl® and Triladyl® (Biovet, France) are commercial extenders containing egg yolk and provide excellent protection for bull semen against freeze shock. Bioxcell® is a commercial extender that contains milk, egg yolk, or both. Gent® A (Minitüb GmbH, Tiefenbach, Germany) is a commercial extender containing egg yolk and is used for the preservation of semen for a long time. EquiPlus® is a commercial extender that contains defined milk proteins used to preserve semen. INRA 96® is a commercial extender that contains a caseinate used to preserve semen.

References

Abdi-Benemar H, Jafaroghli M, Khalili B, Zamiri M.J, Ezazi H, Shadparvar A.A. Effects of DHA supplementation of the extender containing egg yolk and a-tocopherol on the freezability and post-thawing fertility of ram semen. Small Rumin. Res. 2015;130(9):166–170.

Acharya M, Burke J.M, Rorie R.W. Effect of semen extender and storage temperature on motility of ram spermatozoa. ARSci. 2019;8(1):14–30.

Adekunle E.O, Daramola J.O, Sowande O.S. Abiona J.A, Abioja M.O. Effects of apple and orange juices on quality of refrigerated goat semen. J. Agric. Sci. Belgrade. 2018;63(1):53–65.

Allai L, Druart X, Contell J, Louanjli N, Moula A.B, Badi A, El Amiri B. Effect of argan oil on liquid storage of ram semen in Tris or skim milk based extenders. Anim. Reprod. Sci. 2015;160(9):57–67.

Alvarez M, Anel-Lopez L, Boixo J.C, Chamorro C, Neila-Montero M, Montes-Garrido R, Anel L. Current challenges in sheep artificial insemination:A particular insight. Reprod. Domest. Anim. 2019;54(Suppl 4):32–40.

Banday M.N, Lone F.A, Rasool F, Rather H.A, Rather M.A. Does natural honey act as an alternative to antibiotics in the semen extender for cryopreservation of crossbred ram semen? Iran. J. Vet. Res. 2017;18(4):258.

Bhakat, M., T.K. Mohanty, V.S. Raina, A.K. Gupta, P.K. Pankaj, R. K. Mahapatra, and M. Sarkar. 2011. Study on Suitable Semen Additives Incorporation into the Extender Stored at Refrigerated Temperature. Asian-Australatian Journal of Animal Science, 24(10): 1348-1357.

Cueto M.I, Fernandez J, Bruno-Galarraga M.M, Pereyra-Bonnet F, Gibbons A. 196 fertilization rate in superovulated Criolla goats following artificial insemination or natural mating. Reprod. Fertil. Dev. 2018;30(1):238–238.

de Menezes E.B, van Tilburg M, Plante G, de Oliveira R.V, Moura A.A, Manjunath P. Milk proteins interact with goat Binder of SPerm (BSP) proteins and decrease their binding to sperm. Cell Tissue Res. 2016;366(2):427–442.

Fathi M, Zaher R, Ragab D, Gamal I, Mohamed A, Abu-El Naga E, Badr M. Soybean lecithin-based extender improves Damascus goat sperm cryopreservation and fertilizing potential following artificial insemination. Asian Pac. J. Reprod. 2019;8(4):174–180.

Gunawan M, Setiorini S, Fitri H.N, Kaiin E.M. The effect of siam orange juice (*Citrus nobilis* Lour.) in extender on Garut Ram (*Ovis aries* L.) spermatozoa quality post-cryopreservation. J. Phys. Conf. Ser. 2020;1442(1):012068.

Habibi M, Zamiri M.J, Akhlaghi A, Shahverdi A.H, Alizadeh A.R, Jaafarzadeh M.R. Effect of dietary fish oil with or without Vitamin E supplementation on fresh and cryopreserved ovine sperm. Anim. Prod. Sci. 2017;57(3):441–447.

Liu C.H, Dong H.B, Ma D.L, Li Y.W, Han D, Luo M.J, Tan J.H. Effects of pH during liquid storage of goat semen on sperm viability and fertilizing potential. Anim. Reprod. Sci. 2016;164(1):47–56.

Lukusa K. Dietary Supplementation of Selenium and Addition of Vitamin C and E in Extender to Enhance Semen Cryopreservation and Reproductive Performance of Saanen Goats (Doctoral Dissertation, University of Pretoria) 2019.

Manjunath P. New insights into the understanding of the mechanism of sperm protection by extender components. Anim. Reprod. 2018;9(4):809–815.

Masoudi R, Sharafi M, Shahneh A.Z, Towhidi A, Kohram H, Zhandi M, Shahverdi A. Effect of dietary fish oil supplementation on ram semen freeze ability and fertility using soybean lecithin-and egg yolk-based extenders. Theriogenology. 2016;86(6):1583–1588.

Maxwell W.M, Stojanov T. Liquid storage of ram semen in the absence or presence of some antioxidants. Reprod. Fertil. Dev. 1996;8(6):1013–1020.

Mehdipour M, Kia H.D, Nazari M, Najafi A. Effect of lecithin nanoliposome or soybean lecithin supplemented by pomegranate extract on post-thaw flow cytometric, microscopic and oxidative parameters in ram semen. Cryobiology. 2017;78(10):34–40.

Mohamed M.Y, Abd El-Hafeez A.M, Shaarawy A.M. Influence of adding different energy sources to the bull and ram spermatozoa exposed to different refrigerating times. Egypt. J. Sheep Goats Sci. 2019;14(2):1–18.

Nitin Raheja, Sanjay Choudhary, Sonika Grewal, Neha Sharma and Nishant Kumar. 2018. A review on semen extenders and additives used in cattle and buffalo bull semen preservation. Journal of Entomology and Zoology Studies. 6(3): 239-245.

Pankaj, P.K. 2006. Study of critical control points in cryopreservation of bovine semen. Ph.D. Dessertation, Dairy Cattle Breeding Division, National Dairy Research Institute, Karnal. Pankaj, P.K., V.S. Raina, B. Roy, T.K. Mohanty and A.K. Gupta. 2009. Critical control points at the level of collection, processing and preservation of Sahiwal Bull Semen. Indian Journal of Animal Science, 79(10): 992-1000.

Pankaj, P.K., V.S. Raina, B. Roy, T.K. Mohanty and Aditya Mishra. 2009. Effect of Antioxidant Preservative on cold protection ability of low grade riverine buffalo (Bubalus bubalis) bull spermatozoa. Asian-Australatian Journal of Animal Science, 22(5): 626-635.

Prieto-Martínez N, Bussalleu E, Garcia-Bonavila E, Bonet S, Yeste M. Effects of *Enterobacter cloacae* on boar sperm quality during liquid storage at 17 C. Anim. Reprod. Sci. 2014;148(1-2):72–82.

Purdy P.H. A review on goat sperm cryopreservation. Small Rumin. Res. 2006;63(3):215–225. Rahmatzadeh M, Kohram H, Zare Shahneh A, Seifi-Jamadi A, Ahmad E. Antioxidative effect of BHA in soya bean lecithin-based extender containing glycerol or DMSO on freezing capacity of goat semen. Reprod. Domest. Anim. 2017;52(6):985–991.

Rammutla T.L. Effect of Different Disaccharides as Energy Supplements in Tris-Egg Yolk Semen Extender on the Quality of Cryopreserved Boer Goat Spermatozoa (Doctoral Dissertation) 2018.

Sadeghi S, Del Gallego R, García-Colomer B, Gómez E.A, Yániz J.L, Gosálvez J, Silvestr M.A. Effect of sperm concentration and storage temperature on goat spermatozoa during liquid storage. Biology. 2020;9(9):300.

Schulze M, Nitsche-Melkus E, Hensel B, Jung M, Jakop U. Antibiotics and their alternatives in artificial breeding in livestock. Anim. Reprod. Sci. 2020;220(9):106284.

Sukanya R, Phubet S, Srisuwan C, Visid T. Effects of sugar types in semen extender on sperm quality and longevity of frozen goat semen. J. Int. Soc. Southeast Asian Agric. Sci. 2018;24(1):152–161.

Sun L, Fan W, Wu C, Zhang S, Dai J, Zhang D. Effect of substituting different concentrations of soybean lecithin and egg yolk in tris-based extender on goat semen cryopreservation. Cryobiology. 2019;92(1):146–150.

Vidal A.H, Batista A.M, da Silva E.C.B, Gomes W.A, Pelinca M.A, Silva S.V, Guerra M.M.P. Soybean lecithin-based extender as an alternative for goat sperm cryopreservation. Small Rumin. Res. 2013;109(1):47–51.

Zaghloul A.A. Relevance of honey bee in semen extender on the quality of chilled-stored ram semen. J. Anim. Poult. Prod. Mansoura Univ. 2017;8(1):1–5.

18

Synchronization of Estrus in Small Ruminants

S.D. Kharche, Y.K. Soni and S.P. Singh

Division of AP&R, ICAR-Central Institute for Research on Goats Makhdoom, Mathura- 281 122, Uttar Pradesh

Introduction

Goats remain an important and instant source of income as well as livelihood for the majority (70-90 %) of small and marginal farmers in India. Goats are the animals with multiple utility like milk, meat, hide, fibre and manure. They are more tolerant to harsh environment (better resistance to heat stress and drought, better utilization and digestibility of pastures) and give more production per unit investment. Goats are spontaneously ovulating, poly-estrous animals and show seasonal pattern in reproductive activity related to the annual variations of photoperiod. Onset and length of their breeding period throughout the year is dependent on different environmental and physiological factors viz. latitude and climate, feed and fodder availability, breed and breeding system. This in turn affects round the year availability of meat and milk to full fill the market demands. When kids are born out of season, adequate supply of pastures along with good management practices must be ensured in order to minimize kid's mortality and promote their optimum growth.

Estrus induction / Synchronization regimen for cyclic Goats/breeding Season

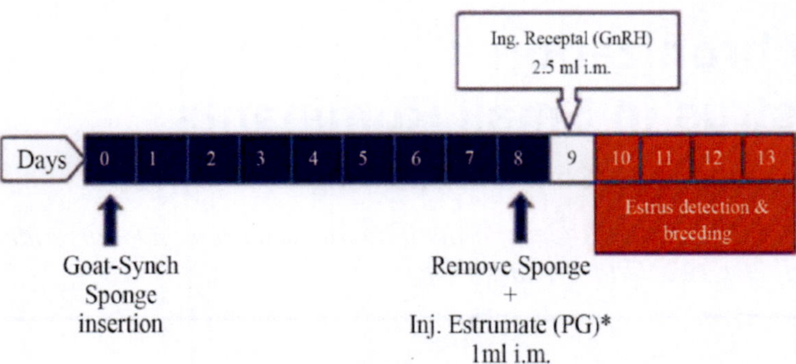

Estrus induction/Synchronization regimen for Anoestrus Goats/Non-breeding Season

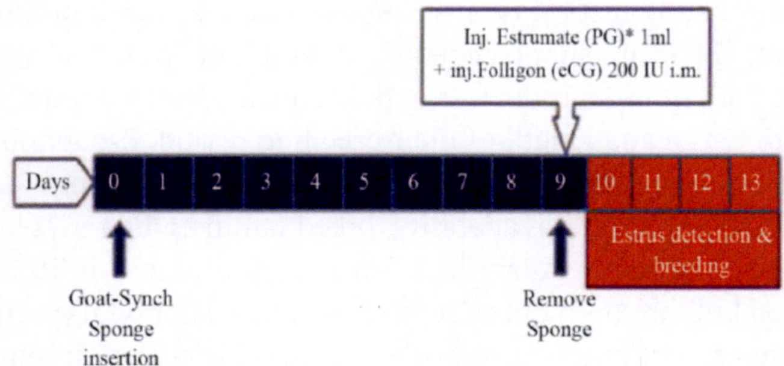

The development of reproductive techniques such as oestrus synchronization is directed to facilitate the genetic improvement of the productive characteristics of the flock and also aimed to speed up the genetic improvements of small ruminants by the increase of offspring of selected males and females and the reduction of the generation intervals. Synchronization of estrus or ovulation is a technique through which most of the females in a flock can be brought to estrus and ovulation at a predetermined time using hormonal or in combination with other management tools. This offers the advantage to group the flock into desired kidding pattern, ensuring uninterrupted supply of meat and milk throughout the year. Furthermore, estrus synchronization reduces the time and labour required for heat detection, allows planned breeding of more number of females at a time and maximizes the use of AI using frozen semen from\ superior sires.

Estrus synchronization is a key element of all the ART protocols in livestock animals and has a major influence to increase the overall efficiencies of these programs. Oestrus synchronization plays a major role in fixed-time breeding, AI, laparoscopic-aided ovum pick-up (LOPU) for oocytes or embryo collection, and Embryo Transfer (ET). This technique has been developed in the early 1960s and since then several synchronizing methods have been developed for sheep and goats. Approaches toward synchronizing oestrus in livestock have to focus on either the manipulation of the luteal or the follicular phase of the estrous cycle. In the doe, the window of opportunity is generally greater during the luteal phase, which is of longer duration and more responsive to manipulation. Different approaches have been concerned with either extending the luteal phase by supplying exogenous progesterone or shortening this phase through regression of the corpus luteum. There are several ways to control the estrous cycle such as light manipulation, the male effect, and hormone treatments with progesterone, prostaglandin (PGF), equine chorionic gonadotropin (eCG), and gonadotropin- releasing hormone (Kharche et al. 2010). Among these hormone treatments, the synchrony of oestrus has been highlighted as a tool to improve the reproductive efficiency of flocks. Successful techniques must not only establish synchrony but also provide a reasonable level of fertility in the synchronized cycle (Rahman et al. 2008). Current approaches to synchronization are classified into pharmacological methods by the use of progestins (MGA, MAP, FGA, vaginal sponges, PRID & CIDR-B), prostaglandins (PGF), and GnRH (Kharche et al. 2010); males' exposure and environmental manipulation.

Estrous cycle of sheep and goats

The knowledge of the estrus cycle is an important aspect before synchronization. It makes it possible to understand the various mechanisms which govern various protocols used during synchronization. The main causes that limit the use, and success of artificial insemination following synchronization are the lack of knowledge of the estrus cycle and poor oestrus detection, which is particularly important in breeds raised under sub-tropical and tropical conditions. The species variation in estrous cycle characteristics is summarized in table 1.

Table 1. The species variation in estruos cycle characteristics.

Animal	Type of estrus cycle	Length of estrus cycle (days)	Duration of estrus	Time of ovulation	Time of insemination
Goat	Seasonal poly-oestrus in Fall	18-21 Average: 19.5	1-4 days Average: 39 hours	21-36 hours after the start of estrus	18 hours after the onset of the heat
Sheep	Seasonal poly-oestrus in Fall	14-20 Average: 17	20-42 hours Average: 30 hours	At or near the end of estrus	12-18 hours after the onset of estrus

Pharmacological Methods Progestins

The breeding season begins when the duration of daylight becomes shorter and ends in winter when the photoperiod is increasing in goats. However, considerable variation exists between goat breeds (Zarazaga et al. 2008). During the mating season, oestrus can be synchronized by intra-vaginal progestogen pessaries, progesterone implants, or prostaglandin. Does show oestrus 36–48 hours after the removal of pessaries or implants. Moore (1980) applied 30 mg FGA in pessaries inserted for around 18 days. A small dose (about 300 I.U.) of PMSG was applied at the time of removal. When a single injection of 100 μg of a prostaglandin analog (EstrumateICI) is used, oestrus occurs one day later and with somewhat less precision than after pessaries treatment.

Out-of-season breeding, Goats in most temperate areas of the world is a short-day breeder with peak breeding activity occurring during late summer, autumn, and early winter (Moore 1980). In tropical regions close to the Equator there is some evidence of polyoestric activity throughout the year (Gonzales Stagnaro et al. 1984) but still more observations are required in these regions. To induce oestrus and ovulation in the anoestrus does progestogen pessaries with PMSG can be used but fertility is dependent upon the stage of anoestrus and time of postpartum treatment (Jackson and Whitley, 2002). In dairy breeds, conception rates at induced oestrus are not high until around one month before the start of full breeding activity and during lactation full fertility is not restored until some three months after kidding (Fonseca et al. 2005). Corteel et al. (1988) described two different treatments to induce oestrus and ovulation in the anoestrus dairy goat; a Long Lasting Progestogen Treatment (LLPT) (45 mg of FGA administered by vaginal sponges for 21 days) associated with PMSG (500–700 I.U.) injected intramuscularly 48 hours before sponge removal. The Short Lasting Progestogen Treatment (SLPT) (45 mg of FGA administered by vaginal sponges but for 11 days) is associated with two intramuscular injections, one of PMSG (500–700 I.U.) and one of cloprostenol (PGF2 analog - 200 μg) both given 48 hours before sponge removal. Fertility based on blood plasma progesterone levels was slightly higher after Short Lasting Progestogen Treatment than after Long Lasting Progestogen Treatment (72.5% vs. 68.2%); kidding percentages were significantly higher, favoring the Short Lasting Progestogen Treatment (62.4% vs. 54.9%); the month of A.I. also had an influence. In Senegal, within the framework of the project of improvement of the Sahelian goat's milk production by the use of AI, we applied the following protocol on 371 does sponge (45mg of FGA) from day 0 to day 11; intramuscular injection of 500 I.U. PMSG and 50 μg cloprostenol on day 9. On day 13, we inseminated does detect in heat (If the does stand still, she was definitely in heat). We obtained a rate of synchronization and conception of 73.32% and 65.2% respectively (Kouamo and Sawadogo 2011). In developing countries, the calendar of reproduction is not established and the control of the breeding is done traditionally. Offspring born out of season, if there are no cultivated pastures available, cannot be grown successfully. The structure of goat production is also quite different in developing countries where the goat flocks are in the hands of nomads and poor goat keepers. So the use of out-of- season breeding needs very good management and a good feed supply; this type of farm is very scarce in developing countries This implies the necessity to combine reproduction improvement programs with pasture improvement and technical assistance.

During the breeding season, only compounds with characteristics identical to progesterone, especially in having a short duration of the activity, are suitable in sheep. When FGA (30 mg) and MAP (60 mg) have been compared in ewes by artificial insemination, a small but significant advantage in favor of FGA was found (Smith et al. 1981). Robinson (1968) mentioned that a progestogen dose that will inhibit ovulation in the cyclic ewe is lower than that required for full fertility. The rate of absorption of FGA from intravaginal sponges can be significantly affected by the impregnation procedure and by the initial dose of the compound (Robinson et al, 1968). The absorption rate significantly affected the percentage of ewes in oestrus and the number of sheep lambing to service at the controlled heats. The procedure currently used for oestrus synchronization during the breeding season is to insert the vaginal progestogen pessaries (MAP or FGA) in the vagina for 14 days, creating an artificial cycle for all ewes. When the pessary is removed ewes will show oestrus 2 to 4 days later. An alternative approach to the intravaginal sponge in sheep is the subcutaneous implant containing the natural hormone, progesterone. According to Gordon (1983) using progesterone implants in Ireland, it has not been possible to match the speed and simplicity of the intra-vaginal sponge technique. The use of progesterone releasing devices associated with eCG or follicle-stimulating hormone (FSH) in oestrus induction/synchronization programs has shown significant effects on oestrus response because gonadotropins stimulate ovarian follicular growth of cyclic or acyclic females (Maurel et al. 2003). Oestrus response and ovulation start earlier and synchronized ovulation is induced when progestagen is associated with eCG (Dogan and Nur 2006). The eCG provides an increase in the diameter of the dominant follicle by acting on the hypothalamic-pituitary-ovarian axis and altering intra-ovarian regulatory mechanisms, besides increasing the maximum diameter and the growth rate of large follicles. Hormonal treatments during the autumn season provide a good level of synchrony of oestrus, resulting in average pregnancy rates of 60% in the first oestrus after device withdrawal. Thus, 90% of cyclic ewes can become pregnant in two natural services that can be performed over 21 days (Moraes et al. 2002). Reproductive efficiencies of the progestogen treatment at various times during the spring season, however, are still variable. Santos et al. (2011) reported that the implementation of the progestogen-eCG hormonal treatment in mixed-breed wool and hair ewes resulted in a considerable oestrus induction/synchronization as measured by a 46% pregnancy rate in the first three days of the mating period. Moreover, the treatment increased the pregnancy rate of mixed-breed wool and hair ewes by approximately 29% points over the controls at the end of the mating season. Thus, the eCG treatment and exogenous progestogen protocol used for oestrus induction/synchronization seem to be a good procedure to be implemented as part of the reproductive management of some ovine farms during the spring season.

Out of season, progesterone implants and progestogen Intra vaginal sponges can be used for oestrus induction in sheep. In most out-of-season applications it is also considered essential to augment the supply of exogenous gonadotrophin by administering a follicle-stimulating agent on completion of the progestogen treatment. The cheapest, most readily available, and consistently effective gonadotrophin for this purpose is PMSG. So ewes may be induced to breed outside their normal sexual season by the combined use of a 12-day progestogen phase to simulate the estrous cycle and an injection of a gonadotrophic hormone, usually PMSG, to cause ovulation. With this method, the ewe shows oestrus 48–60 hr after PMSG (400–700 I.U.) which is injected at the time of sponge or implant removal. Amer and hazzaa (2009) used 40mg of FGA sponges for 6 or 12 days without gonadotropin hormone such as eCG and 40mg FGA sponges for 6 or 12 days and eCG (500IU) to evaluate the effects of intravaginal sponge on the reproductive performance and fertility rate of Rahmani ewes during the anestrous season, found using intra-vaginal

FGA in 12 days with eCG adequate to improve the reproductive performance in the ewes and possible use FGA in 6 days with eCG but fertility are lower. Hashemi et al. (2006) used 20 mg progesterone acetate in oil every day for 12 days, CIDR impregnated (0.3 g P4) for 12 days, and 60mg MAP for 12 days and following intramuscular injection 500 IU eCG, found when used CIDR and MAP give higher effectiveness to oestrus synchronization for ewes. The objective in almost all cases is to advance breeding season to produce early lambs to catch a market premium. This method also could be used to create 2 lambing per year.

Prostaglandin injection

The prostaglandin F2α works by inhibiting the production of progesterone from the ovary. During the normal estrous cycle in the ewe and does prostaglandin F2α is synthesized and released from the uterus, causing the regression of the corpus luteum (Goding 1974). In comparison with the oestrus response after progestogen treatment in ewes and does, the incidence of oestrus that follows the prostaglandin method may be much lower (Kharche et al. 2005); also the fertility rate is depressed. If the natural prostaglandin F2α agent is employed, the accepted luteolytic dose of 15 mg is about 60% of that required in the bovine; using the cloprostenol analog, 100 μg has been employed as a luteolytic dose, which is only 20% that employed in the cow. In comparison with the progestogen or progesterone treatment, the prostaglandin (PG) treatment is more expensive. To use PG the ewe must be in the 5th-13th day of her cycle so that to synchronize, all ewes in the flock, 2 injections are given 9 days apart. Ewes show oestrus on 2–3 days after the second injection. Prostaglandin has also been used as a co-treatment in effective progestogen-based synchronization protocols in sheep and goats for both natural mating and AI/timed AI situations. The use of progestogen or progesterone in combination with eCG and PGF2α usually produces a high rate of oestrus (approaching 100%) even during the transitional period (Kharche et al. 2010). The use of PGF2α or its analogs is considered essential for efficient synchronization in goats (Bretzlaff et al. 1992) since progestogens do not hasten luteolytic processes as in the ewe. Nonetheless, treatment with progestogens without combined administration of prostaglandin may induce luteal regression and oestrus synchronization but extended time is needed (19 to 21 days, compared with 11 to 14 days in ewes). Rubianes et al. (2003) proposed the use of a "short priming protocol" in which ewes and does are treated with progestogen for 5 days and 200–300 I.U. of eCG is administered at sponge/CIDR removal. They reported that the progestogen treatment for longer than 5 days results in sub-luteal concentrations of progesterone that promote excessive growth and persistence of the largest dominant follicle, leading to lower fertility following AI. Using their proposed "short priming protocol" and eCG, a 68% pregnancy rate was achieved following fixed-time AI (54 h from sponge removal) with fresh semen.

GnRH

Ovulation can be synchronized more precisely by administering gonadotropins release hormones (GnRH) around the time of oestrus (Kharche et al. 2008). This improves the success of fixed-time insemination, and the collection of ova/embryos at a controlled stage of development for specific applications of zygotes for pronuclear microinjection (Kharche et al. 1996). The use of pharmacological doses of GnRH in conjunction with intravaginal sponges to induce ovulation was evaluated by Robin et al. (1994) in dairy goats. A single injection of GnRH (125 μg) and a double injection (125 μg/injection in a 48-h interval) at sponge (MAP, 60 mg, 14 d) removal delayed ($P < 0.01$) onset of oestrus and the timing of endocrine events associated with ovulation compared to PMSG-treated does. The pregnancy rate was also lower ($P < .05$) in does receive single and double injections of GnRH than does treat with PMSG (0 and 12% vs 57%, respectively). However, a single injection of GnRH (0.008 mg) at standing oestrus following intravaginal sponge (Progesterone, 300 mg, 12 d) and PMSG treatment increased the pregnancy rate (66.67 vs 70.42%) in Jamunapari goats (Kharche et al. 2010). In Merino ewes treated with GnRH injection (100 μg) 24 h after sponge removal (MAP, 12 days), the time to ovulation was advanced in the breeding season, but the treatment did not affect the timing of ovulation in the anoestrus season (Ryan et al. 1992). Similarly, shortening of the time to onset of oestrus was observed in cyclic Merino when GnRH (100 μg) was injected 12 h after sponge removal (MAP, 12 days; Jabbour and Evans 1991). It seems doubtful that bolus injections of GnRH can stimulate ovulation to the same extent previously seen with sustained GnRH treatment protocols.

Male exposure

Estrus can be induced with the strategic exposure of anoestrus does and ewes to intact males or androgen treated castrates. This response is dependent on the depth of seasonal anoestrus and associated with the first ovulation in 2 to 3 days. Exposure to males after a period of isolation can be used for induction and synchronization during the breeding and non-breeding season without additional treatments in goats. Does lactating in the fall due to summer breeding was used to compare the effect of no treatment (buck exposure during the breeding period only) to temporary kid removal (48h) after approximately

28 days of lactation. Although temporary kid removal decreased days to first mating compared with does still nursing kids, all does were bred within 10 d after the introduction of bucks and there was no influence of treatment on kidding rate (79.0 ± 0.1%), average birth weight (3.3 ± 0.2kg), or weaning weight of removed or subsequently born kids (Fletcher et al. 2002). Hence, kid removal was not necessary to synchronize lactating does during the breeding season (Whitley and Jackson 2004). Research conducted by Romano (1994a) suggested that the duration of oestrus was reduced when bucks were allowed to service the does, as opposed to merely mounting the does, and that this response was mediated through the mechanical action of the penis against the vagina (Romano 1994b). Certain authors suggested the incorporation of the male effect into oestrus synchronization. The "ram effect" (the ability of the odor of the ram to induce oestrus) in anoestrus ewes may be used to replace injection of PMSG; ewes must have been isolated from rams for at least 4 weeks. The ram is introduced on the day the vaginal sponge is removed (Umberger et al. 1994). Another combination treatment consists of implants of melatonin in conjunction with the "ram effect" (Croker et al. 1988). Only effective during the breeding season, PG use (in combination with the male effect) may still offer a flexible, economical method for synchronization to shorten the breeding season in a natural mating situation. The 'ram effect'and 'buck effect' combined with progestogen treatment, have also been used to induce early breeding in flocks of ewes and does during the non-breeding season.

Environmental manipulation

Controlled lighting is used routinely to regulate the onset of sexual maturity in pullets and regimes have been devised to stimulate earlier initiation of ovarian activity in seasonal breeding mammals. Sheep and goats are influenced by photoperiod to be autumn breeders, a characteristic that is accentuated in environments of great photoperiodic variation. In sheep and goats, photoperiod allows by stimulating the secretion of hormones, the hypothalamus GnRH and pituitary gland LH, effects on reproductive function (Duygu and Köker 2011). Light treatment to alter photoperiod response is a well-known synchronization method for out-of-season breeding in the dairy goat industry. However, time and housing constraints may be impractical for commercial meat goat producers. Administration of melatonin to mimic altered photoperiod may be an effective alternative (Whitley and Jackson 2004). The manipulation of the breeding cycle in ewes can be done also by artificial day length control (Gordon 1983). It can be a matter of providing a gradual decrease or increase in artificial day length, similar to what occurs under natural day length conditions or it may be done by subjecting the ewes to an abrupt decrease on one day and thereafter maintaining them at that day length until a response is shown (Fraser and Laing 1969). One partial disadvantage in using day length control is the fact that individual ewes show oestrus after varying intervals; several weeks may elapse between the time the first and the last sheep in the flock comes on heat. This system requires electrification of the rural areas. Moreover, certain photoperiodic treatments may change the speed of hair growth and light treatment during pregnancy was shown to delay about 4 weeks the onset of puberty in young female goats born from light-treated mothers (Deveson et al. 1992b).

References

Amer HA and Hazzaa AM. 2009. The effect of different progesterone protocols on the reproductive efficiency of ewes during the non-breeding season. Veterinarski Arhiv. 79 (1):19-30.

Bretzlaff KN, Nuti LC, Elmore RG, Meyers SA, Rugila JN, Brinsko SP, Blanchard TL and Weston PG. 1992. Synchronization of oestrus in dairy goats given norgestomet and estradiol valerate at various stages of the estrous cycle. American Journal of Veterinary Research 53, 930-934.

Corteel JM, Leboeuf B and Baril G. 1988. Artificial breeding of goats and kids induced with hormones to ovulate outside the breeding season. Small Rumin. Res. 1, 19-35.

Croker KP, Johns MA and Staples LD. 1988. Use of regulin melatonin implants in conjunction with teasing of Merino ewe flocks joined in Spring. Proc. Aust. Soc. Reprod. Biol. 20, 75 (abstr.).

Deveson S, Forsyth IA and Arendt J. 1992. Retardation of pubertal development by prenatal long days in goat kids born in autumn. J. Reprod. Fertil. 95(2), 629-37.

Fletcher CM, Jackson DJ and Whitley NC. 2002. Use of 48-hour kid removal to decrease the post-partum rebreeding interval in meat does. J. Anim. Sci. 80 (Suppl1.): 290. (Abstr).

Fonseca JF, Torres CAA, Costa EP, Maffili VV, Carvalho GR, Alves NG and Rubert MA. 2005. Progesterone profile and reproductive performance of estrous-induced Alpine goats given hCG five days after breeding. Animal Reproduction Science 2 (1): 54-59.

Fraser AF and Laing AH. 1969. Oestrus induction in ewes with standard treatments of reduced natural light. Vet. Rec. 84, 427–430.

Goding JR. 1974. The demonstration that PGF2α is the uterine luteolysin in the ewe. J. Reprod. Fert. 38, 261-271.

Gonzalez-Stagnaro C, Blanc M, Pelletier J, Poirier JC, Poulin N, Fagu C, Baril G and Corteel JM. 1984. Variaciones de la secretion de FSH, LH y progesterona durante el celo natural o inducido en cabras alpinas. Proceed. Xth Intern. Cong. Anim. Reprod. Artif. Insem. 3, 325.

Hashemi M, Safdarian M and Kafi M. 2006. Estrous response to synchronization of estrus using different progesterone treatments outside the natural breeding season in ewes. Small Ruminant Research 65: 279-283.

Jackson DJ and Whitley NC. 2002. Effectiveness of melengestrol acetate in inducing out-of-season breeding in goats. J. Anim. Sci. 80 (Suppl.2), 29 (Abstr).

Kharche SD and Srivastava SK. 2005. Synchronization of oestrus and subsequent conception in dairy cows treated with prostaglandin F2 α. Indian J. Anim. Science 75 (8) :932-933.

Kharche SD, Goel AK, Jindal SK and Sinha NK. 2008. Birth of a female kid from in vitro matured and fertilized goat oocytes. Indian Journal of Animal Sciences 78(7): 680- 85.

Kharche SD, Singh N, Goel AK and Jindal SK. 2010. Induction of oestrus and fertility following insertion of intravaginal pessaries in anoestrus Jamunapari goats. In Proc.: International conference on Biotechnologies for optimization of reproductive efficiency of Farm companion animals to improve global food security% human healthand 26th Annual convention of ISSAR, GBAUAT, Pantnagar, 11-12th November, 2010, pp. 141.

Kharche, S. D., Goel, A. K., Jindal, S. K. and Sinha, N. K. 2005. Efficacy of Crestar Ear Implant for Oestrus Synchronization and Superovulation with PMSG and FSH- P in goats. In: Proceedings XXI Annual Convention of ISSAR and National Symposium on Recent Trends and Innovations in Animal Reproduction, November 23- 25, 2005 at Sher-e-Kashmir University of Agricultural Sciences and Technology, Jammu. pp. 95.

Kouamo J and Sawadogo GJ. 2011. Enzymatic and electrophoretic profiles of serum proteins of the inseminated Sahelian goats in Senegal. Third life science and animal production conference, CAFOBIOS, Dschang, 26-68 may, Cameroon (Personal communication).

Maurel MC, Roy F, Herve V, Bertin J, Vaiman D, Cribiu E, Manfredi E, Bouvier F, Lantier I. Boue P and Guillou F. 2003. Immune response to equine Chorionic Gonadotropin used for the induction of ovulation in goats and ewes. Gynecol. Obstet. Fertil. 31, 766-769.

Moore NW. 1980. Procedures and results obtainable in sheep and goats. In current therapy in Theriogenology. Ed. D.A. MORROW and W.B. SAUNDERS, 89-95.

Moraes JCF, De Souza CJH and Gonçalves PBD. 2002. Controle do estro e da ovulação em bovinos e ovinos. In: Gonçalves, P.B.D.; Figueiredo, J.R.; Freitas, V.J.F. (Eds.) Biotécnicas aplicadas à reprodução animal. São Paulo: Varela, 2002. p.25-55.

Rahman ANMA, Abdullah RB and Wan-Khadijah WE. 2008. Estrus Synchronization and Superovulation in Goats: A Review. Journal of Biological Sciences 8, 1129-1137.

Romano JE. 1994a. Effect of service number on estrus duration in dairy goats. Theriogenology 41, 1273-1277.

Romano JE. 1994b. Effects of different stimuli of service on estrus duration in dairy goats. Theriogenology 42, 875-879.

Rubianes E, Menchaca A and Carbajal B. 2003. The pattern and manipulation of ovarian follicular growth in goats. Anim. Reprod. Sci.78, 271–287.

Ryan JP, Hunton JR and Maxwell WMC. 1992. Time of ovulation in Merino ewes superovulated with PMSG and FSH-P. Reprod. Fertil. Dev. 4, 91-97.

Santos GMG, Silva-Santos KC, Melo-Sterza FA, Mizubuti IY, Moreira FB, Seneda MM. 2011. Reproductive performance of ewes treated with an estrus induction/synchronization protocol during the spring season. Anim. Reprod. 8, 3-8.

Smith PA, Boland MP and Gordon I. 1981. Effect of type of intravaginal progestagen on the outcome of fixed-time artificial insemination. J. Agric. Sci. Camb. 96, 243–245.

Umberger SH, Jabbar G and Lewis GS. 1994. Seasonally anovulatory ewes fail to respond to progestogen treatment in the absence of gonadotropin stimulation. Theriogenology 42, 1329-1336.

19

Artificial Insemination Techniques in Goats

Ravi Ranjan, Chetna Gangwar and Manish Kumar

Division of AP&R, ICAR-Central Institute for Research on Goats, Makhdoom Mathura- 281 122, Uttar Pradesh

The selection of breeding bucks in relation to maximizing the reproductive efficiency depends upon males. AI permits intense selection of sires with exceptional merits and provides opportunity to exploit the value of superior sires. Young males can be trained for exhibiting sexual behaviors and semen collection through the uses of male, anoestrus doe or oestrus doe as dummy. Successful AI depends on precise management of semen collection, its frequency and use. The semen collection implies mounting a teaser doe or a dummy. Artificial vagina (AV) and electro-ejaculator (EE) are the two methods for semen collection in bucks. AV method is being used as universal method for routine semen collection whereas electro-ejaculation is generally used for collecting semen from untrained and valuable sires incapable of service. Moreover, this method of collection is painful for the animals. Semen evaluation should be rapid and effective so that collected semen samples can be processed for initial quality which ultimately affects the fertility. There are several tests for the assessment of semen quality but no single test is reliable to give definite prediction of the fertility.

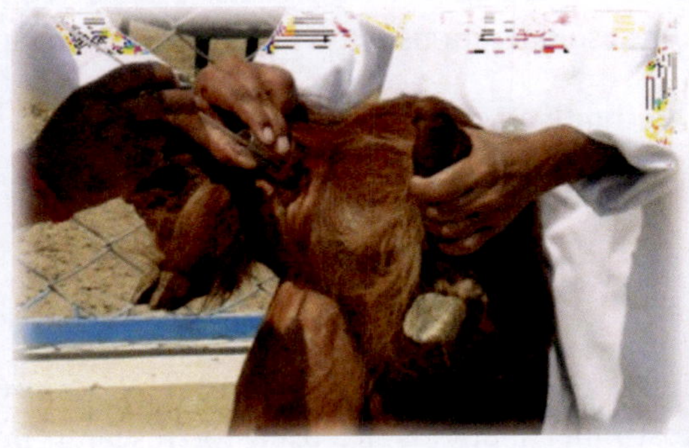

It is said that centuries ago Bedouin horse breeders stole semen of famous stallions by inserting a sponge into the vagina of a mare before service and then successfully transferring the sponge to their own mares. The first documented use of artificial insemination of domestic animals was done by the Italian

Physiologist L. Spallanzani in 1780. A new landmark in the field of AI was established in 1949, when Polge et al., (1949) discovered a practical method for the long time preservation of semen of certain species by deep freezing to temperatures of -79^{0}C by means of dry ice (CO_2).

AI. is the deliberate introduction of semen into a female reproductive tract for the purpose of achieving a pregnancy through fertilization by means other than mating/ natural service.

In India, A.I. in goats is relatively less developed as compared to cattle and buffaloes. The main reason is being lack of realization of the economic importance of goats.

Human population will be reach to 1.7 billion and goat population will be 216 million by 2050 (ICAR-CIRG, Vision 2050). Therefore, to meet requirement of milk, meat and associated by products of ever-increasing human population, it is imperative to increase goat productivity. It could be possible by increasing high productive descript (33%) goat population and reducing non-descript (67%) and less productive goats by promoting scientific goat farming. There are 71 million breed able does and 17 million breeding bucks available in India as per 12th Livestock Census Report. One buck by natural mating can cover maximum 50 does in a year, but by stored frozen semen 3000 does can be covered in a year. Therefore, to cover 71 million breed able does, we need 1.5-2 million bucks as compared to only 50,000 bucks needed for Frozen Semen AI Technology. Artificial Insemination (AI), is the first generation of reproductive biotechnology by which we can replace the non-descript and less productive goats with productive goat population. AI and semen cryopreservation represents a pivotal tool for the long-term ex-situ in vitro conservation, exchange of valuable germplasm of livestock and endangered species. Encouraged by the experimental work on AI in goats, several A I Centers and Veterinary clinics in different parts of the country have started by maintaining 2-4 stud goats. The mixed AI centers would reduce the cost of these operations. However, few centers are operating exclusively for goats.

Methods of AI

1. Intravaginal
2. Intracervical
3. Intrauterine

Intravaginal and Intracervical AI is mainly used by most of workers. The rest other methods are used for research purpose. For Intra cervical AI, the oestrous goat lifted from back for clear visualization of genitalia. A lubricated glass vaginal speculum is inserted through vagina for visualization of cervical opening under sunlight. Then fresh or frozen thawed semen straw inserted through vaginal speculum and go through cervical opening and semen was deposited there and waits for two to three minutes. Clitoral massage should be done for better fertility. AI should be done twice at 12 hours interval. If a goat come in oestrous in morning, then AI should be done in evening of the same day and morning of the next day.

There is complex cervical anatomy in goats having 3-6 cartilaginous cervical folds and are horizontally aligned. It is very difficult to pass the AI gun throughout the cervix. So, the conception rate highly correlated with depth of penetration. This technique is more suited in goats and easy to perform. The total time taken is 2-3 minutes. The pregnancy rate is 20-55% (FAO, 2012).

AI equipment and supplies

1. Carrying case
2. Kit warmer
3. Artificial insemination (AI) gun
4. AI gun sheaths
5. AI light
6. Vaginal speculum
7. Straw tweezers
8. Straw cutter
9. Non-spermicidal, sterile lubricant
10. Semen thaw unit
11. Insemination reports
12. Fresh Cooled or Frozen Semen
13. Vaginal Swabs
14. Liquid Nitrogen Storage Tank

Factors affecting AI

The success of any AI program is largely dependent on three primary factors:

1. The use of live/viable fresh cooled or frozen semen.
2. The appropriate timing of insemination in relation to estrus and ovulation.
3. The proper deposition of semen in the doe.

Other factors affecting AI

1. The breed
2. Age of buck and doe
3. Condition of buck and doe
4. Nutrition
5. Season of insemination
6. The use of fresh, cooled, chilled, frozen semen
7. The technical/labour involved
8. Time of insemination
9. The extender used Dose of inseminated semen
10. The method (vaginal, cervical, cervicouterinal or laparoscopic) used

Fertility with frozen semen

Although the laparoscopic AI involving deposition of frozen-thawed semen directly in to the uterus generally results 60-70 % fertility (Salaman et al., 1995), the conception rate of cryo-preserved semen following trans-cervical AI (TCAI) is still very low (16-40 %; Kumar et al. 2014). The premature capacitation as a consequence of freezing and thawing curtails the lifespan of spermatozoa having very shorter time to achieve fertilization compared to the fresh sperm. Therefore, further research efforts are required to develop better freezing protocols and diluents that minimize the ultra-structural and biochemical alterations in spermatozoa resulting from the freezing/ thawing process, particularly if intended for TCAI; because spermatozoa have to survive longer to traverse through cervical mucosa before reaching the site of fertilization. The kidding rate was 37.57% during 2016-17 at this Institute in four breed of goat Jamunapari, Barbari, Jakhrana and Sirohi through Frozen Semen AI Technology.

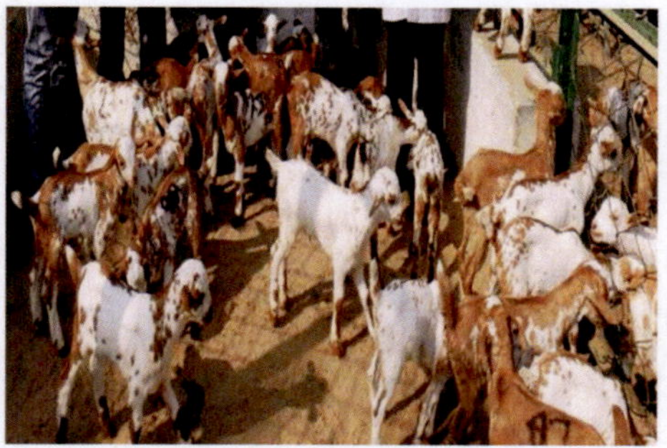

Applications

The pioneering work on technique in goat carried out at Indian Veterinary Research Institute, Izatnagar and Veterinary College, Mathura revealed around 50% conceptions after first insemination with washed spermatozoa diluted in EYC diluents. Though the attempts of AI in goats have been undergone on experimental basis at various organized farms and Research Institution of India, still serious and coordinated efforts are lacking for taking up the AI in goats on large scale like AI in cattle and buffaloes. Research work on freezability of buck semen with the use of citrate-yolk milk and tris-citrate acid yolk diluents was carried at veterinary college Anand, Guwahati, Tirupati, Ranchi, Bombay, Akola, NARI and Mathura including Central Institute for Research on Goat (CIRG), irrespective of glycerol percentage (3-9%) and equilibration time (0-6 hrs.), post-thaw motility varied between 42-66 %. There was71.43% pregnancy rate with kidding rate of 1.27 by pellet semen. Conception rate was poor (35-45%) due to deposition of frozen semen over the opening of cervix. Improvement in fertility (55-65%) was observed due to deep cervical insemination technique.

Important application of AI

1. The technique helps to introduce a new or desirable genotype into the livestock population at a faster rate.
2. High quality semen produced by superior sires can be used to breed large number of does.
3. AI helps in genetic management.
4. The maintenance of a large number of males, which would otherwise be required, is reduced.
5. Al permits reproduction when suitable males are not available for natural mating.

6. The technique provides accurate breeding records for good herd management.
7. AI improves the efficiency of on-farm progeny testing schemes by a better elimination of the flock effect.
8. Valuable sires which are incapable of mating due to age or injury may be utilized through electric ejaculation.
9. AI prevents stray mating and also solves the problems of mating of animals of unequal size.
10. The technique helps control disease transmission, since males used for insemination are under health control and do not circulate from one flock to another.
11. The technique can be used as a means of sex control through separation of X- and Y- spermatozoa before use.
12. Artificial insemination has been used experimentally to yield hybrids between species that do not voluntarily mate.

Limitations

1. There is possibility of dissemination of hereditary defects or uncontrolled diseases.
2. Lack of awareness on the part of goat keepers of the economic advantages of using selected progeny tested males.
3. Conception rate with AI is lower than that of natural mating.
4. Due to lack of cheap and practical technique of oestrus synchronization in the tropical goats, the farmer has to spend lot of time in heat detection and breeding operations. Lack of interest on the part of concerned agencies to encourage the concept of mixed AI centres (cow, buffalo and goat) which is quite feasible in the existing AI setup in India.
5. Illiteracy among farmers, religious taboos and sentiments also serve as limiting factors.
6. There is a need for arranging short visits of scientists for exchange of experience, discussions and mutual understanding of problems of fundamental and applied nature in AI of goats.
7. A sound programme does not exist for training of extension workers in AI of goats at the national and provincial level.

20

Laparoscopic Artificial Insemination in Small Ruminants

Y.K. Soni, S.P. Singh and S.D. Kharche

Division of AP&R, ICAR-Central Institute for Research on Goats Makhdoom Mathura- 281 122, Uttar Pradesh

Artificial Insemination (AI) is one of the most popular first generation assisted reproductive technology as well as a breeding tool, ever evolved for the genetic improvement of cattle and buffalo industry throughout the world. The advent of frozen semen has further revolutionized this technique. Presently, use of sex- sorted-semen in cattle breeding is also coming into vogue. Contrary to cattle and buffalo, use of AI in small ruminants has not gained such impetus.

It has been reported that lower pregnancy rates were obtained when ewes and does are bred with frozen or extended liquid semen using intra-vaginal or intra-cervical technique of insemination. The reason being anatomy of the cervix of sheep and goats; cervix is long and tortuous with presence of 4-7 cervical rings. Furthermore, these cervical rings are directed caudally hindering the lumen of the cervix thereby causing hindrance (more prominent in sheep) while passing the AI gun during intra-cervical or trans-cervical AI (TCAI). There are several reports which support the fact that, as the depth of semen deposition into the cervix increases, the pregnancy rates also improve due to availability of a greater number of motile sperms for fertilization.

Laparoscopic Artificial Insemination (LAI)

Laparoscopic Artificial Insemination (LAI) is an advanced assisted reproductive technique that involves deep intra-uterine deposition of frozen or extended semen into the reproductive tract of small ruminants (sheep and goats), bypassing the anatomical barrier of cervix. This technique is based on the principles of minimal access surgery by using laparoscope.

Consistently higher pregnancy rates (60-80%) were reported using LAI as compared to conventional intra-vaginal insemination or TCAI. Moreover, lower sperm concentration can be used per LAI which further maximizes the use of breeding males. The average dose required for breeding a ewe using frozen semen can be as less as 20-25 million live spermatozoa, when compared to higher doses required for intra-vaginal (nearly 400 million live spermatozoa) and TCAI (100-200 million live spermatozoa).

The main disadvantage of LAI is high equipment cost and requirement of surgical expertise to perform the procedure safely. However, with the availability of newer and more portable laparoscopy equipment, it is now possible to offer these services cost-effectively at a hospital and field setting.

Materials required

- 5mm Trocar and Canula: 5mm (2 no's)
- Veress needle (one)
- 5mm 0° Telescope/endoscope
- Light source/Fibre optic cable
- Video camera and monitor screen
- Insufflation port and tube
- LAI cradle
- Sterile laparotomy surgical pack
- Trans cap with guide (IMV, France)
- Aspics for semen straws
- Semen straws (0.25ml)
- Straw cutter
- Lint free paper towel
- Semen thawing unit
- Slide warmer
- Microscope for semen evaluation
- Suture material (catgut 1-0, cotton thread, traumatic and atraumatic needles)
- Anesthetics (Ketamine, Xylazine, Lignocaine)
- Injectable antibiotics, anti-inflammatory, anti-histaminic

Procedure of Laparoscopic AI

Selection of animal

- Although the technique of LAI is minimally invasive, still healthy females of appropriate body condition score (BCS-between 2 to 4) are the most suited candidates for this technique. Animals with optimum BCS are reported to have higher ovulation as well as pregnancy rates.
- Obese animals are not fit for any laparoscopic procedure in small ruminants because;
- Excessive fat interferes with the laparoscopic instruments; hence visualization of reproductive tract becomes difficult.
- Abdominal fat exerts excessive pressure on diaphragm causing hypoxia to patient in Trendelenburg position.
- Obese animals may not respond to estrus synchronization protocols. This may be due to increased clearance of the steroid hormones from systemic circulation because of increased liver blood flow, thereby reducing their bioavailability.
- Animals should be properly vaccinated, dewormed and free from any kind of systemic illness.
- While applying estrus synchronization protocols, thorough knowledge about reproductive physiology, seasonal and breed variations and drug dosage.
- A thorough knowledge of reproductive physiology, seasonal and breed variations, appropriate duration of protocols and drug dosages are essential for adequate response.

Estrus detection

Animal must be in proper heat before the actual procedure of LAI. Heat detection should be carried out by parading aproned teaser buck twice daily as per AM-PM schedule along with visual signs of estrus; wagging or fanning of tail (most reliable sign), swollen vulva, bleating and seeking males etc.

Preparation of animal

- Keep the animal off-fed for at least 16-20 h or one day before LAI and off-water for at least 12 h. This reduces the content of bladder and rumen, which may interfere in locating, and viewing of uterus. It also avoids regurgitation and aspiration during laparoscopy.

- Procedure room should be clean, dust free and a sterile place.
- Pre-medication and preparation of animal should be done in room just outside the procedure room.
- It must ensure that the animal has passed the urine before the LAI; it minimizes the accidental injury to urinary bladder.
- Clean shave the area of the abdomen just 10-12 cm anterior to udder.
- Any visible dirt, dung etc. around the procedure site should be washed using Savlon or mild soap and wipe it dry using sterile gauge.
- Light sedation is usually recommended since the total duration of the procedure (preparation and surgery) ideally takes roughly about 10-15 min only. The goal is to have the patient stand up on their feet within few minutes just after the procedure.
- Inj. Xylazine@ 0.05 - 0.1 mg/kg body weight of the 20 mg/ml large animal formulation I.V. or I.M.
- After that immediately take the animal in the laparoscopy room and restrain in dorsal recumbency on a specially designed laparoscopy cradle.
- Adjust the cradle at an angle of 45^0 so that animal comes in head down (Trendelenburg position).
- Now, firmly secure all the four legs of animal on four ends of cradle using rope.
- Scrub the shaved area using 70% isopropyl alcohol or Betadine antiseptic solution.
- Now, infiltrate Local anesthetic, 2ml of 2% lignocaine hydrochloride subcutaneously 7-8cm (a palm width) anterior to the udder and 3-4 cm each side of the mid ventral line adjacent to the left and right mammary/ superficial epigastric veins.

All the instruments to be used in the laparoscopic procedures must be sterilized and be ready to use and must be easily accessible to surgeon. In back-up, one sterilized surgical pack must be ready for laparotomy in case of any kind of accidental damage to internal organs or to check internal bleeding.

Exploratory laparoscopy

- Now make two small (2cm) incisions with angular surgical blade No 11, in the skin approximately 4-6 inches in front of the udder, one on each side of midline avoiding blood vessels and linea alba.

- Insert the 5mm trocar and canula through left side by gentle, consistent and calculated pressure in drilling action (hold the trocar and canula just like a pistol and close the opening of trocar by thenar eminence just below the base of the thumb).
- Keep the direction of trocar-canula slight lateral to avoid puncturing the visceral organs.
- As soon as the abdominal wall gets punctured a click sound will be felt that confirms the correct positioning of port.
- Now remove the trocar, leaving the canula in its place.
- Now insufflate the abdomen to create pneumoperitoneum using Co or filtered air to maintain the pressure around 6-8mmHg with flow rate 5lit/min.
- Pneumoperitoneum can be created prior to insertion of trocar-canula using 14 cm Veress needle to avoid injury to internal organs and blood vessels by trocar.
- Ensure that abdomen is tensed enough to visualize the abdominal organs and should not cause any respiratory distress to the animal.
- Insert 0 degree, 5mm Hopkins type, straight rigid endoscope (Karl Storz, Germany) through this port and visualize the reproductive organs.
- Urinary bladder is used as landmark to locate the reproductive organs which can easily found on either side of the bladder.
- Once reproductive organs are visualized, make another incision just opposite to previous one and insert second 5mm trocar-canula.
- In case reproductive organs are not visible, insert a palpation probe through this second port to manipulate the organs in the field of vision.
- Now remove the trocar leaving canula in its place. Loading of LAI gun and insemination
- Loading of semen straw (0.25ml) into aspic is very crucial and should be done carefully.
- Frozen semen is thawed at 37^0C for 30 seconds and wiped with lint free tissue paper.
- Straw is cut and loaded from the back side of aspic and gently fixed with red coloured plunger/stick.
- Now remove the needle cap from aspic and insert into the guide.

- Keeping the needle tip within the guide, now introduce this loaded gun into abdomen.
- Guide can be used to manipulate the horns, if not properly visualized so as to expose uterine horns.
- After proper positioning put the tip of guide over the avascular part of greater curvature and give quick thrust with needle to penetrate into the lumen.
- With the help of assistant push the plunger/rod (Red stick) of trans cap so as to deposit the semen into the uterine horns.
- Half of the semen can be deposited into another horn.
- Observe that the factory plug of semen straw should reach at the tip of the aspic which confirms successful insemination.
- Fine blood spot can also be observed that indicates successful puncture.
- Now withdraw the gun as well as laparoscope and release the air completely from the abdomen.
- Close the skin incisions by single stich using non-absorbable suture material (cotton thread etc.).
- Pour local antibiotics and dress the suture sites using Betadine or any other ointment.
- Gently, unload the animal from the cradle and administer anti- histaminic, anti-inflammatory and long-acting antibiotics.
- Observe the animal daily for 3-5 days and remove the sutures after one week. Pregnancy can be diagnosed as early as 35 days post-insemination using real time B-mode ultrasonography.

21

Methods of Pregnancy Diagnosis in Goats

S.P. Singh, S.D. Kharche and Y.K. Soni

Division of AP&R, ICAR-Central Institute for Research on Goats, Makhdoom Mathura- 281 122, Uttar Pradesh

An early and accurate diagnosis of pregnancy is a crucial factor for successful management and maintaining cost-effective production in scientific goat production for better economic returns. In addition, accurate information on the stage of gestation would also be useful to dry off lactating females at an adequate period. The techniques for pregnancy diagnosis in goats are mostly depend upon visualization of the conceptus or determination of its secretory products in the maternal blood or the milk are the most defined and specific methods for pregnancy. The choice of pregnancy diagnosis method in goats depends on the stage of gestation. Some methods have a higher degree of accuracy at the early gestation while others do at the late stage of gestation. Assessment of pregnancy in terms of hormonal assay of blood plasma, serum, or milk, and estimation of pregnancy-specific antigens or proteins give a higher level of accuracy within 30 days of pregnancy. There are many methods that are currently being used for pregnancy diagnosis in goats. Among those, the method applied should be safe for both offspring and mother and need to be low-cost and easy to apply. Various techniques have different kinds of limitations to their wide-scale use. These techniques are classified into 3 classes, which are as follows:

1. Visual methods
2. Clinical methods
3. Laboratory tests

1. Visual methods

Non-return to oestrus: At the point when the mated animal does not come back to oestrus, the standard presumption is that the animal is pregnant and subsequently has not come back to oestrus. This happens during pregnancy because conceptus restrains regression of corpus luteum and thus prevents the animal from returning to oestrus. Conversely, many time animal does not return to the oestrus in view of non-regression of CL because of reasons other than pregnancy. In addition, in the seasonally breeding species animals may not return to the oestrus because the season is over.

Other visual methods: In addition to the non-return to oestrus other visual signs of pregnancy diagnosis in late pregnancy include an increase in the size of the abdomen, development of the udder, slightly vaginal discharge, and movements of the fetus visible externally but the accuracy of these visual diagnostic symptoms always low and the clinician must use them as a complement to clinical diagnosis.

2. Clinical methods

Clinical methods of pregnancy diagnosis include rectal palpation abdominal ballottement, radiography, ultrasonography, and laparoscopy.

Rectal palpation: Pregnancy diagnosis in large ruminants such as cattle and buffaloes by transrectal palpation is the oldest and most widely used method. It is the easiest, most economical and fastest method for early pregnancy diagnosis with little or nil harm to the animal. Rectum palpation in goats and sheep is of no value because of the size of the pelvis. Rectal abdominal palpation, in which a glass rod is inserted in the rectum to lift the uterus which is palpated through the abdomen, is suggested for goats and sheep. Likewise, bimanual palpation (palpation of the uterus through fingers in the rectum and lifting the abdomen) is also reported in small ruminants. The fetus is palpated through the abdominal wall by moving the stick side-to-side. This method is reliable after 50 days of gestation.

Abdominal ballottement and abdominal palpation: Abdominal palpation is feasible in goats and sheep only beyond 4 months of pregnancy by lifting the abdomen held between both hands.

Radiography: Radiography is used for pregnancy diagnosis to a limited extent in small ruminants (sheep and goats). This technique is fast; around 400 to 600 ewes can be diagnosed per day under farm conditions. In sheep and goats, fetuses are visible by day 70 of growth with high precision. The overall accuracy of this technique in detecting pregnancy increases with advancing gestation: 52% between 66 and 95 days to 100% following 96 days. The exactness of determining fetal numbers approaches 87% just between days 91 and 110. In this manner, radiography is proposed to be done simply after day

90 in sheep and goats. In addition, the high cost and the hazards of exposure to developing fetuses to X beams restrain the utilization of radiography as a normal methodology and warrant its utilization in particular cases.

Ultrasonography

Three main types of ultrasonographic systems are usually used for pregnancy diagnosis in the small ruminants

a) **A-mode ultrasound (Amplitude-depth or echo-pulse)**: it is a quick, convenient and simple technique but still it cannot predict the fetus number and viability of fetuses. In this framework, the transducer emits ultrasound waves that penetrate tissues under the skin and are reflected when meeting high acoustic impedance interfaces (pregnant uterus or liquid-filled structures). The transducer gets the reflected echoes and changes over them into the peaks on the oscilloscope with a horizontal scale representing the depth of the reflecting structure or into an audible signal. Meredith and Madani (1980) utilized reflection of ultrasound at a depth of 9 cm or more noteworthy as a positive indication of pregnancy in ewe and announced 96 % sensitivity and 87.5 % specificity in the period from 61 to 151 days after mating.

b) **Doppler ultrasound:** Doppler devices use the Doppler Principle to identify the fetal heartbeats and stream of blood in uterine and fetal vessels. The intrarectal Doppler system could be utilized for diagnosing pregnancy at the start of the second trimester with an accuracy of 90% or better. The accuracy of the intra-rectal Doppler transducer for diagnosing pregnancy and non-pregnancy was 82% and 91% respectively, from days 41 to 60 of gestation. After day 71 accuracy ranged between 85 to 94% for the same.

c) **Real-time, B-mode ultrasonography:** Real-time B-mode ultrasonic scanning of the uterus in small ruminants seems to offer an accurate, quick, protected, and practical means for diagnosing pregnancy, determination of fetal numbers, and estimating gestational time.

Laparoscopy

Laparoscopy can be utilized as a strategy for pregnancy diagnosis by directly visualizing the genitalia in animals. The invasive nature of the technique, the high cost of equipment and clinical required, and the accessibility of non-invasive techniques limit the utilization of this method as a method for pregnancy diagnosis in goat and sheep

3. Laboratory test

The different laboratory tests produced for pregnancy diagnosis in domestic animals are indirect techniques for pregnancy assessment, and use qualitative or quantitative measures of reproductive hormones at particular stages after AI or mating, or recognize conceptus particular substances in maternal body parts or body liquids as an indicator of the presence of a viable pregnancy.

Progesterone test

Estimation of blood progesterone concentration is an important indicator of the functional corpus luteum. The concentration of plasma progesterone samples was measured in ewes at day 18 post-breeding by utilizing enzyme immunoassay (EIA) and radioimmunoassay (RIA). The accuracy of these assays for determining pregnancy was high, while it was low to diagnose non-pregnancy.

Estrone sulfate test

The estrone sulfate is formed by the feto-maternal axis or the conceptus and consequently, its presence in urine, milk, feces, or blood is an indicator of pregnancy. The detection of estrogens relies upon the accessibility of appropriate laboratories and accessibility of commercial assay kits. Laboratories evaluating the concentration of estrogens in urine or serum are usually equipped with radioimmunoassay, enzyme Immuno-assay, or other more accurate and particular diagnostic modalities for the measure of steroids in urine, serum, feces, or other body liquids.

Caprine placental lactogen (caPL)

The caPl are purified and commercialized by numerous labs. Radioimmunoassay of caPL accomplished 97 and 100 % accuracy for diagnosing pregnant and non-pregnant ewes at day 64 of growth, respectively.

Pregnancy proteins

A highly polymorphic family of placenta-expressed proteins was discovered in the ruminant species. These pregnancy-associated glycoproteins (PAGs), also known as pregnancy-specific protein B (PSPB) and pregnancy serum protein (PSP). These proteins are used as pregnancy markers due to their site of origin i.e. mono- and bi-nucleate cells of placenta. The use of specific antisera allowed the discrimination between pregnant and nonpregnant goats as early as 21 days after breeding.

PAGs are potential biomarkers in early pregnancy in goats. PAGs are structurally correlated to aspartic proteinase and are expressed in the outer epithelial cell layer (trophectoderm) of the placenta. They have been found to share about 50% amino acid sequence identity with pepsinogen, pepsin, cathepsin D, and cathepsin E.

PAG enzyme-linked immunosorbent assay

Recently, a sandwich kind of enzyme-linked immunosorbent assay (ELISA) is developed and utilized to recognize PAG concentration in blood plasma and milk samples of goats (Singh et al., 2019a; 2021). For this, a mixture of peptide-based antibodies raised against semi-purified PAG molecules was used/ The concentration of PAG, which was measured by ELISA, increased gradually between Days 24 and 45 of pregnancy (Singh et al., 2018). Moreover, the capacity of this assay to differentiate pregnant and non-pregnant females, as well as single and multiple fetus-bearing does in early gestation was also evaluated (Singh et al., 2019a, 2019b).

Conclusion

Early and accurate detection of pregnancy and the number of fetuses in goats is an important factor in improving the reproductive efficiency of animals and achieving high economic output. In recent years, multiple methods for pregnancy detection in small ruminants with varying degrees of precision and accuracy have been developed and evaluated. Each method has benefits and disadvantages based on their results and eases to perform the test. Few of them are invasive or of low accuracy hence of limited practical use in the field conditions. Others are precise but require equipment and specialized skills. The practical implementation of user-friendly, on-farm, accurate and non-invasive methods for pregnancy detection in goats compatible with animal welfare standards would result in optimization of the reproductive performance.

22

Disease Transmitted Through Artificial Insemination in Goats

K. Gururaj, A.K. Mishra, Anu Rahal, Nitika Sharma, R.V.S Pawaiya, Ashok Kumar and D.K. Sharma

Division of Animal Health, ICAR-Central Institute for Research on Goats Makhdoom, Mathura- 281 122, Uttar Pradesh

Introduction

Artificial Insemination is a very important tool that caters to propagation of high-quality germplasm and breed improvement. It is also economical as it aids in breeding without the necessary to maintain the adult bucks cutting the input cost. However, the bucks maintained for production of semen and AI should be free of any diseases and in specifically venereal diseases. Venereal diseases are not so uncommon in livestock, and they cause a variety of symptoms including orchitis, abortions, still birth, vulvovaginitis etc., leading to infertility in breeding animals. Venereal diseases are infectious in nature and they are transmitted mainly through semen, feed-water, AI gun, artificial vagina, fomites etc. Due to venereal diseases, infertility, orchitis, epididymitis, vasculitis etc. occurs in bucks and leads to abortions and still birth in does (Ahmed et al, 2010; Beena et al, 2017), because they are directly linked with the economic output (Sharma et al, 2008; Azawi et al, 2010) and overall health of the animal affecting the productivity significantly (Menzies, 2011). To keep abortions and other venereal diseases at bay, it is important to raise disease free breeding bucks that deliver clean-semen for natural service or AI operation. Abortion rate between 2 to 5% indicates its endemic nature and abortion level exceeding 5% requires aggressive investigation (Menzies, 2011). Infectious agents that include viruses, bacteria, fungi, parasites etc.; as well as non-infectious cause can lead to infertility in goats (Moeller, 2001; Szeredi et al, 2006; Smith and Sherman, 2009). Many infectious causes are known to mankind that leads to trans-venereal diseases in goats including *Brucella melitensis*, Chlamydiosis, *Campylobacter* spp., *Listeria monocytogenes*, Toxoplasmosis, *Coxiella burnetii* etc. There are numerous viruses such as

Akabane, Cache Valley, Blue Tongue, Border Disease, Herpesvirus, Nairobi Sheep Disease, PPR, Rift Valley Fever, Wesselsbron Disease, Bovine Viral Diarrhea etc, which are capable to cause caprine abortions (Smith and Sherman, 2009). Under viral agents, caprine herpes virus is the most common one in causing abortions in goats (Moeller, 2001; Kahn and Line, 2010). Most of these infectious agents are also of zoonotic importance since the aborted materials usually contain huge number of these organism excreted in it and the exposure of these infectious agents also pose a very high occupational risk to farmers, animal handlers and veterinarians. Parasitic agents such as *Toxoplasma gondii*, *Neospora caninum*, *Sarcocystis*, *Anaplasma* etc. may cause abortions in goats (Smith and Sherman, 2009; Shaapan, 2016). Among parasitic agents, the most common agent is *Toxoplasma gondii* (Smith and Sherman, 2009; Kahn and Line, 2010; Shaapan, 2016). The fungal agents associated with the abortions are *Aspergillus, Candida, Mucor, Rhizopus, Penicillium, Cladosporium, Rhodotorula, Absidia, Alternaria* and *Fusarium* (Pal et al, 1985; Pal, 1988; Verma et al, 1999). Aspergillus followed by Candida is the most prevalent fungi associated with abortion in goats (Vandyousefi and Zoghi, 1988 and Munoz et al, 1989). The bacteria and bacteria related microorganisms causing abortion in goats are *Brucella, Chlamydia*, *Coxiella burnetii*, *Campylobacter*, *Listeria monocytogenes*, *Leptospira* (mostly interrogans, grippotyphosa and pomona), Mycoplasma, Salmonella, *E. coli*, *S. aureus, Pseudomonas aeruginosa, Streptococcus, Aeromonas, Fusobacterium, Trueperella pyogenes* etc. (Moeller, 2001; Szeredi et al, 2006; Sharma et al, 2008; Smith and Sherman, 2009; Menzies, 2011). The most common bacteria and bacteria related microorganisms causing caprine abortions are *Brucella melitensis, Chlamydophila, Coxiella burnetii and Listeria monocytogenes* (Sharma et al, 2008; Menzies, 2011; Rossetti et al 2017; Rajagunalan et al, 2019). The aborted materials such as placenta, foetus, vaginal discharge etc. generally contain large number of the infectious agents and the exposure of these agents may pose a very high occupational risk to farmers, animal handlers, veterinarians etc. Hence, while handling these materials, we should follow strict biosafety measures. In the current chapter, we will discuss about the major abortogenic infectious agents in goats.

Brucellosis (Contagious Abortion)

Brucellosis is highly zoonotic disease-causing abortion and infertility in livestock, resulting in severe economic loss to livestock owners. Brucellae are usually species specific affecting a wide range of host from domestic to wild animals and marine mammal and there are nine identified *Brucella* spp. that are classified based on host and antigenic variation. This includes *B. melitensis* (host - Sheep and goats), *B. abortus* (host- cattle), *B. ovis* (host- Sheep), *B. suis* (host- Pigs), *B. neotomae* (host- Wood rats), *B. canis* (host- Dogs), and

B. microti (host- Common voles). In human, it is also called Undulant fever, Malta fever, Gibraltar fever, Mediterranean fever, Mediterranean remittent fever; in animals - contagious abortion, abortus fever, infectious abortion, epizootic abortion and Bang's disease. Brucellosis in goats caused by *Brucella melitensis (B. melitensis)*, and rarely by *B. abortus* or *B.suis.* The major cause of abortion in small ruminants is brucellosis and it affects the reproductive tract sometimes leading to infertility. The major clinical feature of brucellosis is retention of placenta, orchitis and epididymitis, arthritis, and the major public health hazard is the excretion of the *Brucella* spp in discharges and milk of Brucella infected animal. *Brucellae* are coccobacilli or short rods, non-motile, gram-negative, moderate acid-fast aerobic bacteria. Seroprevalence of the disease ranges from 3 to 18 % in goats of India. The organism is facultative intracellular parasite of the reticuloendothelial system. The bacterium gets entry mainly through the mucous membranes of the oropharynx, upper respiratory tract, eyes and male or female genital tract. It is also transmitted through intact skin, wounds and artificial insemination. Aborted foetal content or foetal membranes, vaginal exudates and milk are potential sources of the infection. Following the infection, the organisms multiply in the chorionic epithelia resulting in inflammation, degeneration, autolysis and necrosis of the epithelia, which results abortion. The disease causes abortion in late pregnancy. Clinical signs include retention of placenta, metritis, mastitis in females and orchitis, epididymitis, osteoarthritis, infertility and synovitis in males. Brucellosis is a zoonotic disease; humans may get infected with this disease either through consumption of infected milk or handling during kidding. Diagnosis of the disease is usually made by isolating the organism from foetus, placenta, vaginal discharges or milk. ELISA, PCR, agglutination, precipitation, and complement fixation tests are commonly used to detect the carrier goats. An allergic skin test (Brucellin test) can be used as a screening test to identify infected goats. World-wide, most prevention and control programmes focused on bovine brucellosis and to some extent it has been eradicated or controlled, but ovine-caprine brucellosis was less addressed and it still remains a major problem in the goats and sheep. One of the significant attributes to this problem is the under reporting of the incidence of caprine brucellosis from the field conditions mainly due to lack of validated and standardized caprine-specific diagnostic assays; and then the widely used serological tests for screening brucellosis in cattle were not effectively standardized for use in small ruminants. Hence, diagnostic tests with high specificity are required for diagnosis of brucellosis in small ruminants mainly caused by *B. melitensis*, which is also incidentally the most common cause of human brucellosis in India. Besides serum tube agglutination test (SAT) and iELISA, there are a variety of options available for screening of brucellosis in goats including bruce-ladder PCR, AMOS PCR, OMP25, *OMP2* based RFLP (Gupta et al. 2012) and OMP31 gene based conventional and Real time probe-based PCR (Saini et al. 2017). However, it is always better to rely on more than one test to arrive at the confirmatory diagnosis (Gupta et al. 2014).

Treatment of brucellosis is difficult because the organism is an intracellular parasite. Long-acting oxytetracycline (25 mg/kg I/M every 2nd day for 28 days) combined with streptomycin (20 mg/kg I/M every 2nd for 14 days) may be useful. Vaccination of kids and lambs three to six months of age with *B. melitensis* Rev 1 vaccine (live attenuated) is recommended universally for prevention of the disease. Frequent sero-screening program in goat herds should be implemented and sero-positive goats must be slaughtered immediately as per "test and slaughter" policy.

Chlamydiosis

Chlamydiae are involved in various clinically important diseases in cattle, sheep and goats including abortions and stillbirth with predominant lesion being placentitis, urogenital diseases, conjunctivitis, pneumonia and polyarthritis. Members of the order Chlamydiales are ubiquitous, obligate intracellular gram-negative organisms that contain both RNA and DNA. Earlier, the organism was known as psittacosis lymphogranuloma venereum trachoma agent, *Miyagawanella* and *Bedsonia*. In 1999, genera *Chlamydia* and *Chlamydophila* were proposed for the members of the order Chlamydiales but now, it is no longer valid. Presently, a single genus, *Chlamydia*, is used which consists of 11 species namely *abortus*, *caviae*, *felis*, *muridarum*, *pecorum*, *pneumoniae*, *psittaci*, *suis*, *trachomatis, avium* and *gallinacea*. Transmission of the disease from animal to man is well known for *C psittaci*, *C abortus* and *C felis*. Likewise, chlamydial species of man (*Chlamydia trachomatis*) has been detected in numerous animal species. Chlamydial infections in goats are responsible for arthritis, keratoconjunctivitis, respiratory diseases and most important one, abortion. The organism only replicates in intracellular location competing with the host for intracellular nutrients. That is why; it cannot be grown on an artificial medium. It has two forms during its life cycle as elementary body which is infectious in nature, and reticulate body which is a metabolically active non-infectious form. The infectious elementary bodies (EB) are shed through feces, nasal, ocular or vaginal discharges and uterine fluids or aborted fetus are potential reservoirs that can transmit to healthy animals of the herd. In affected animals, microscopically there is necrosis of trophoblastic epithelium with infiltration of neutrophils. The available methods for diagnosis are staining, immunohistochemistry, ELISA etc. However, more efficient ways of diagnosis can be molecular based detection techniques such as PCR and real-time PCR using 16srRNA and IGS-S genes as targets.

Abortion in goats is caused by *Chlamydia abortus.* In many areas, chlamydial abortion is the second cause of infectious abortions after brucellosis and the main cause where brucellosis is controlled. The abortion is generally seen during the last months of pregnancy with stillbirths or premature births of weak kids with low birthweight. The abortion affected doe generally does not show clinical signs, and the placenta is usually not retained. Fertility of the does usually remains normal after the subsequent abortions. Infected doe excretes a large number of *Chlamydiae* in placenta and fetal fluids at the time of kidding and abortion. *Chlamydiae* may come in vaginal fluids for a period of two weeks before, and after abortion. *Chlamydiae* gain access to fetus and placenta through intestine, genital tract and conjunctiva. The placenta of aborting does is very precious for diagnosis of the chlamydiosis. Presumptive diagnosis of the disease can be done by demonstration of elementary bodies in impression smear using special stains such as Giemsa, Stamp, Macchiavello, modified Ziehl-Neelsen etc. The confirmatory diagnosis can be done by isolation of the organism in cell culture or in embryonated eggs, ELISA, IFT, CFT, PCR etc. Oxytetracycline (long acting; @ 20 mg/kg of body weight on every 3rd day) or tylosin (orally; 20 mg/head/day) significantly reduce outbreaks of chlamydial abortions. For prevention of occurrence of chlamydial abortions, all biological materials associated with the abortion (fetus, placenta, fluids etc.) should be removed, and properly disposed off. The concerned area should be made sterile. The aborting females should be separated for several weeks until they stop shedding *Chlamydiae.* Contamination of feed and water with the soil must be avoided.

Coxiellosis

Coxiellosis is also called Q fever, Queensland fever, Query fever and Abattoir fever because the cause of an outbreak of illness (fever) amongst abattoir workers in Queensland, Australia was not known at that time (year 1935). Dr. Burnet identified *Coxiella burnetii* (*C. burnetii*) as cause of illness in 1*937. Coxiella burnetii* is the obligate intracellular rickettsial organism which is pleomorphic (coccoid to short rod), weakly acid-fast and variably Gram-negative and it has been reported in five continents viz., Africa, America, Asia, Europe and Oceania except New Zealand with zero prevalence. In nature, *C.*

burnetii exists in virulent form (Phase I), whereas in embryonated eggs or cell cultures, it is found as less virulent Phase II form. Like other rickettsial organisms, it cannot grow non-living medium. Coxiellosis is a zoonotic disease, and can be used as a potential biological warfare agent because it is very infectious and highly stable in the environment as well as capable of windborne spread. Cattle, sheep and goats are the primary reservoirs of *C. burnetii*. The prevalence of *C. burnetii* was reported slightly higher in cattle compared to the small ruminants, but with lack of well-designed studies no reliable data on prevalence available. However, it can infect wide variety of animal species such as dogs, cats, rabbits, horses, pigs, camels, buffalo, rodent, birds etc. The organism is shed heavily in placenta, birth fluids, colostrum, milk, urine and feces. Abortion or stillbirth in goats due to coxiellosis occurs mostly in late pregnancy without prior clinical symptoms. The abortion due to *C. burnetii* infection in goats is generally not seen, however, there are many investigations in which abortion rates were reported up to 90%. Reproductive problems associated with the infection usually do not relapse following the abortion. Inhalation is the most common route of entry of the organisms in to animals as well as humans. The agent is shed in high numbers during parturition and in aborted materials contaminating the environment, this massive contamination of the paddock with the organism excreted during abortions can facilitate oral transmission of the agent. The resistance of the agent to various environmental factors and disinfectants along with aerosol spread increases the risk of infection to humans. Dairy goat flocks were also an important source of infection for humans. Aerosolized *C. burnetii* bacteria can move up to 11 miles. In addition to inhalation, the spread may occur via ingestion, tick bite, transstadial and transovarial transmission Decreased immunity amongst the animals, overcrowding, lack of hygiene, virulence of *C. burnetii* etc. may lead to the spread of the infection within the flock/herd. In abortion or stillbirth caused by Q fever, there will be severe damage of placenta with presence of abundant exudate. *C. burnetii* is very dangerous organism, and for its handling, BSL-3 conditions are required. Its identification through microscopy can be done by Ziehl–Neelsen, Gimenez, Stamp, Giemsa and modified Koster stainings. PCR including the *IS1111*gene nested trans-PCR, multiple-locus variable-number tandem repeat analysis, multispacer sequence typing, single nucleotide-polymorphisms, indirect immunofluorescence test, ELISA, micro-agglutination and complement fixation tests can be employed for diagnosis of coxiellosis. Tetracyclines may be tried in flocks or herds aborting due to *C. burnetii*. Q fever abortion can be prevented by adopting good managemental practices, and providing optimum nutrition to the animals.

Toxoplasmosis

Toxoplasma gondii is a protozoan parasite, which is responsible for abortion, mummification, stillbirth, and birth of weak young kids and lambs in goats and sheep, respectively. Cats act as the definitive host (Buxton, 1998), and they become infected by consuming uncooked meat, rodents (Dubey, 1986). The infected cats then shed oocysts in their feces, and this shedding may continue from 3 to 19 days. The oocysts can survive in moist and shaded soil up to 1.5 years (Frenkel, 1982). Toxoplasmosis affects all the warm blooded animals including humans, and is known as a major cause of abortions in sheep since 1950s. Toxoplasma was identified in a classical triad of symptoms viz.hydrocephalus, retinochorditis and encephalitis in children. The oocysts of Toxoplasma gondii shed from cat faeces are a potential source of infection for domestic livestock, pets and human beings. In cats, there is an sexual cycle confined to the enteroepithelial cells producing oocycts, but the asexual cycle comprises of two developmental stages viz., Tachyzoites and bradyzoites. Goats may become infected by eating grass, hay, feed etc. contaminated with feces of the cat. *Toxoplasma* may remain encysted in the muscle, brain, liver etc for years or whole life of the infected goat. If, the goats are infected in their first half of pregnancy, abortions generally result with the dead fetuses. Abortions and neonatal mortality occur in sheep and goats suffering with primary infection. Before abortions, the ewes/does can show febrile pyrexia with rectal temperature as high as 41^{0}C. The tachyzoites invade the caruncular septa of the placentome, invading the trophoblast cells of fetal villi progressing to abortions. Abortion can occur in early, mid and late gestations. The early gestational toxoplasmosis is usually fatal to the dam and can cause infertility. While mid-gestational abortion initiated by toxoplasma leads to mummified fetus, and late abortions leads to fetal mortality, still born lambs/kids or birth of weak neonates. Fetal serology is a very specific test for abortive toxoplasmosis. Generally, absence of antibodies in the does at time of abortion indicates that toxoplasmosis is not the cause of abortion. A modified direct agglutination test (MAT) is considered to be very sensitive, and may be used for diagnosis of toxoplasmosis. Sabin-Feldman dye test, indirect haemagglutination test, indirect immunofluorescent antibody test, latex agglutination test etc. can be used for diagnostic purposes. The disease is highly zoonotic and warrants careful handling of the aborted foetuses' and infected animals. Diagnosis can be made on the basis of serological tests, staining of placental impression smears, Immuno-histochemistry of placental sections, nested single tube PCR for detection of *T. gondii*.

Treatment of the infected goats during pregnancy can be tried with monensin at the normal anticoccidial rate, that is, 20 grams/ton of goat-feed. Deco quinate can be given at dose rate of 2 mg/kg bodyweight for treatment. To prevent occurrence of the disease in goats; contamination of feed, fodder, water etc. with cat-feces must be avoided. Toxoplasmosis is zoonotic disease; hence, human beings may get infection by consuming raw/uncooked meat or milk of goats. Hence, milk and meat should be consumed after pasteurization and proper cooking, respectively.

Listeriosis (Circling Disease/Silage Disease/Caprine Bacterial Encephalitis)

Listeriosis is an important infectious disease of goats most commonly associated with neurologic signs, but also capable of causing septicemia, mastitis and abortion. This disease is of zoonotic importance, and caused by *Listeria monocytogenes,* a motile, aerobic and facultative anaerobic, small, gram-positive bacterium. Milk and meat are the potential sources of the infection for humans. Rise in body temperature (106°F), abortion in late gestation, dullness, depression, pressing of head with wall or some hard surface, unilateral facial paralysis, circling movements in either direction, conjunctivitis with corneal opacity etc. are clinical signs observed in affected animals. Listeriosis in animals arises mainly from the ingestion of contaminated food and water, and is particularly common in animals fed on silage. It is zoonotic in nature and has potential risk of causing food poisoning in humans. The septicemic form of listeriosis leads to abortions in domestic animals. The bacterium *Listeria monocytogenes* causes the disease and it is present in farm ecosystem including soil, feces, nasal secretions, water trough and animal feeds like silage. In goats, the disease is manifested in three forms viz. abortion, encephalitis and septicemia. Septicaemic form is more common in young kids, while abortions occur in the last trimester in sheep and goats. The disease resembles with salmonellosis due to gastroenteritis like symptoms with necropsy lesions including haemorrhage and ulceration/erosion of abomasal mucosa with the duodenum showing congestion. Microscopically, the intestine mucosa will reveal infiltration of neutrophils within the lamina propria. Isolation of the organism, PCR, ELISA etc. are commonly used methods for the diagnosis of the disease. Diagnosis can be made by gram positive staining appearing as small, motile, non-sporulating coccobacilli in cultures made by UVM (University of Vermont medium I and II) and black colonies on Palcam agar. Quick detection can be made from clinical samples using conventional PCR directed against biofilm and virulence associated genes like *prf*A, *plc*A, *act*A, *hly*A and *iap.* In the encephalitic form, intravenous sodium penicillin at a dose of 40,000 IU/kg every 6 hours until improvement is noted, followed by a seven-day course of intramuscular procaine penicillin at a dose of 20,000 IU/kg twice a day is recommended for the treatment. Dexamethasone given once a day at a dose of 0.1 mg/kg intravenously increases overall efficacy of the treatment. Poor quality silage with a pH more than 5 should not fed because it favours the growth of *Listeria monocytogenes.*

Leptospirosis

The other names of the disease are Autumnal fever, Cane cutter's disease, Canicola fever, Harvest fever, Infectious jaundice, Mud fever, Rice field worker's disease, Seven-day fever, Swamp fever, Swine herd's disease, Walter fever, Weil's disease. Leptospirosis is a contagious and zoonotic disease caused by the bacteria of the genus *Leptospira*, and affects humans as well as animals including goats. *Leptospira* is a spirochaete of the family Leptospiraceae, and motile, aerobic, flexuous, helically coiled bacterium ranging from 6-20 μ in length. There are two species of the genus Leptospira namely *Leptospira interrogans* (*L. interrogans*) and *L. biflexa*. *L. interrogans* is a pathogenic species whereas, *L. biflexa* is saprophytic. *L. interrogans* has many serovars capable of causing illness. Various serovars of *L. interrogans* have been isolated from the leptospirosis in goats, most notably *L.pomona, L. grippotyphosa,L. icterohemorrhagiae* and *L.serjoe. Leptospira* most commonly gains entry through penetration of wet skin or mucus membranes of the host. Goats may also get infection by the ingestion of feed and water contaminated with urine from the infected animals. Warm, moist and wet conditions favour the growth of the organisms. The bacteria can survive in the standing water for long periods. Infection causes bacteremia and septicemia then subsequent localization of the organisms in the kidney leading to leptospiremia. Transplacental movement of the bacteria may cause abortion in second half of pregnancy. Fever (104-106°F), anorexia, depression, tachycardia, icterus of mucus membrane, petechial hemorrhages on the conjunctiva and reddish-brown urine are the main clinical signs observed in the disease. In acute leptospirosis, the affected animals without treatment may die within 2-3 days. The organism can be best isolated from blood, kidney and urine. The most practical method for diagnosis of the disease is the assessment the antibody titers in acute and convalescent serum samples taken seven to ten days apart in clinically affected goats The microscopic agglutination test (MAT) is most frequently used test for assessing the antibody titers. This test measures both IgM and IgG antibody, and is mainly useful for the diagnosis of acute leptospirosis than its chronic form. A titer of 1: 300 or more is considered positive for the acute form. A combination of streptomycin and penicillin has been found very effective in treating caprine leptospirosis. A single intramuscular injection of 25 mg/kg of streptomycin may clear the bacteria from the kidney. In place of streptomycin, a single intramuscular injection of long acting oxytetracycline at a dose of 20 mg/kg BW may be tried. Fluid therapy is recommended to maintain water and electrolyte balance, and blood transfusions should be applied in case of the acute anemia. Rodent control, removal of standing water/damp bedding, quarantine, vaccination and screening or prophylactic treatment of newly acquired animals for elimination of the carrier state are the steps to be followed to prevent the disease occurrence. New born kids must be fed with colostrum within 12 hours post birth for acquiring passive immunity. Little or no protective cross immunity occurs among the various serovars of *L. interrogans*, so multivalent vaccines should be used. Kids older than three months of age should be vaccinated, and revaccination at 6-month interval is recommended. Farmers, herders, veterinarians, milkers and slaughterhouse workers are prone to get infections due to their occupations, so they should be very conscious while handling the infected goats/goat-carcasses.

Campylobacteriosis (Vibriosis)

The disease is also called vibrionic abortion or vibrionic enteritis, and is caused by members of genus-*Campylobacter* consisting of a number of species, of which *Campylobacter fetus* subsp. *fetus* (formerly *Vibrio fetus intestinalis*), *C. jejuni*, and *C. coli* are the pathogenic ones. Both *Campylobacter fetus* subsp *fetus* and *C. jejuni* are the common cause of abortion in sheep whereas, campylobacteriosis is less often documented a cause of abortion in goats. Vibrionic abortion in goats is commonly caused by *C. jejuni,* and less frequently by *C. fetus*. Campylobacters are zoonotic, microaerophilic, slender, spirally curved rods with a polar flagellum at one or both ends, and require approximately 10% CO_2 and 3-6% O_2 for their growth. Campylobacters are widely distributed in nature with most of their species adapted to intestinal tracts of warm-blooded animals and birds. The infection can be transmitted by (i) ingestion of contaminated water and feed (ii) direct contact with carriers (human and animals) (iii) sexual contact. Aborting does usually show no clinical signs but may have mild diarrhea and mucopurulent vaginal discharge. Aborted kids may have grossly visible liver necrosis. The placenta is often edematous with necrosis of cotyledons. Confirmatory diagnosis of campylobacteriosis is done by the isolation of the organism which requires specific media and special microaerophilic culture technique. Fetal lung, abomasal content and vaginal discharge are the preferred samples for the isolation of the organism. In addition to this, various immunological and molecular techniques are available for the diagnosis of the disease. In case of an undiagnosed abortion, administration of tetracycline (long acting; 20 mg/kg every 48 hours) may be effective not only against campylobacteriosis but also against several other abortion causing bacterial agents. In case of tetracycline resistant pathogens, sulfamethazine (110 mg/kg orally) or tyrosine (30 mg/kg I/M once daily) may be given. Sanitation at the farms is the necessary step for prevention and control of *Campylobacter* infections. Fecal contamination of feed and water should be avoided and the aborting does should be isolated. Like other abortions, placentas, body fluids and fetuses should be burned or buried deeply. In conclusion, various scientific reports probably indicate that the disease is of minor importance in goats, although of public health significance.

Sampling considerations with special reference to brucellosis: Special care should be taken while sampling for screening and diagnosis of abortigenic agents due to their zoonotic risks associated with them. For Brucellosis, serum can be collected and used for a battery of diagnostic tests including colored plate agglutination test, standard tube agglutination tests, indirect ELISA, 2-mer tests etc. Another way is antigen detection using molecular tests like PCR and Real time PCR targeting various genes from samples like placenta, genital swabs, fetal tissue and contents. Breeding males should be periodically screened for presence of brucellosis before every breeding season which would eventually reduce the abortion storms at farm level. ICAR-CIRG accepts sera, blood, genital swabs for regular screening and diagnosis of suspected animals all over the country for brucellosis. To ease the logistics associated with icepacks and other complications, we have developed a genital swab based TaqMan® probe real time PCR for quick diagnosis of brucellosis in small ruminants. For conducting this test, it requires a sterile cotton swab collected from vaginal mucosa/ preputial mucosa sealed in zippered covers sent through envelope without ice or any preservative to ICAR-CIRG. Alternatively, blood can be collected in filter papers within 1cm diameter circular area dried, sealed in zippered polythene covers with silica desiccant and can be sent to ICAR-CIRG by speed post. The dried blood will be eluted and assayed for IgG iELISA based detection of brucellosis. Care should be taken to properly label and segregate the samples while sending to ICAR-CIRG for efficient communication of results without any confusion. By this it is easier to cater to the whole country where goat keepers who can't access diagnosis can avail such facilities in addressing the brucellosis. Similarly, the genital swabs were also used for screening of other non-brucella organisms such as *Coxiella burnetii*, *Campylobacter*, *Chlamydia*, *Mycoplasma* etc. by PCR based diagnostics.

Conclusion

Besides these listed diseases there are a number of infectious diseases caused by fungal, bacterial, viral and protozoal origin that are transmitted through semen. The epidemiological incidence depends on the geo-climatic zone and the favourable conditions for the spread of a particular disease through semen. Semen, whether frozen or chilled also influences the viability of certain pathogens like Listeria grows well even under frozen conditions for a long period of time. The presence of cryo-protectants in LN2 frozen semen collaterally protects the infectious agents also. Hence it is important to pre-screen the semen for total bacterial and fungal load by Plate count technique based on the prescribed protocol. This should be followed by use of robust efficient, quick and accurate diagnostic techniques to screen the semen for AI or screen the bucks prior to collection of semen.

References

Ahmed, B.H., Hamad, R.J. and Abdelghafar, R.A. (2010) Ultrasonography for diagnosis of hydrometra and pyometra. Assiut Vet. Med. J., 56: 124.

Azawi, O.I., Al-Abidy, H.F. and Ali, A.J. (2010) Pathological and bacteriological studies of hydrosalpinx in buffaloes. Reprod. Domest. Anim., 45(3): 416-420.

Beena V, Pawaiya RVS, Gururaj K, Singh DD, Mishra AK, Gangwar NK, Gupta VK, Singh R, Sharma AK, Karikalan M, Kumar A (2017) Molecular etiopathology of naturally occurring reproductive diseases in female goats, Veterinary World, 10(8): 964-972.

Doley S and Nekibuddin A (2017). Isolation and antibiogram of aerobic bacterial pathogen associated with respiratory tract of apparently healthy goats. International Journal of Chemical Studies, 5 (3): 817-819.

Goat Medicine (2009). Smith MC and Sherman DM (Eds.). Wiley-Blackwell Publication, Iowa (USA), Second Edition.

Gupta, V.K., Nayakwadi, S., Kumar, A., Gururaj, K., Kumar, A. and Pawaiya, R.S., 2014. Markers for the molecular diagnosis of brucellosis in animals. Adv. Anim. Vet. Sci, 2(3), pp.31-39.

Gupta, V.K., Vohra, J., Kumari, R., Gururaj, K. and Vihan, V.S., 2012. Identification of Brucella isolated from goats using Pst I site polymorphism at Omp2 gene loci. Indian Journal of Animal Sciences, 82(3), p.240.

Mahdi AA, Al-Naqshabendy AA and Haddel BT (2015). A study of some pathological lesions in the lung of sheep and Duhok abattoir. Basrah Journal of Veterinary Research, 14 (2):265-277.

Menzies PI (2011). Control of important causes of infectious abortion in sheep and goats. Veterinary Clinics Food Animal Practice, 27: 81-93.

Moeller Jr RB (2001). Causes of caprine abortion: diagnostic assessment of 211 cases (1991–1998). Journal of Veterinary Diagnostic Investigation, 13 (3): 265-270.

Pal M, Mehrotra BS, Dahiya SM (1985). Studies on mycotic abortion caused by Aspergillus fumigatus Fresenius. Indian Journal of Animal Reproduction, 6: 43-48.

Pal, M (1988): Aspergillus niger associated with mycotic abortion in buffalo (Bubalus bubalis). Mycoses, 31: 17-19.

Rajagunalan S, Gururaj K, Lakshmikantan U, Murugan M, Ganesan A, Sundar A, Sureshkannan S, Andani D, Pawaiya RS. Detection of the presence of Coxiella burnetii in a case of goat abortion: a first report from India. Tropical animal health and production. 2019 May 1;51(4):983-6.

Rossetti CA, Arenas-Gamboa AM, Maurizio E (2017). Caprine brucellosis: A historically neglected disease with significant impact on public health. PLoS neglected tropical diseases, 11(8).

Saini, S., Gupta, V.K., Gururaj, K., Singh, D.D., Pawaiya, R.V.S., Gangwar, N.K., Mishra, A.K., Dwivedi, D., Andani, D., Kumar, A. and Goswami, T.K., 2017. Comparative diagnostic evaluation of OMP31 gene based TaqMan® real-time PCR assay with visual LAMP assay and indirect ELISA for caprine brucellosis. Tropical animal health and production, 49(6), pp.1253-1264.

Shaapan RM (2016). The common zoonotic protozoal diseases causing abortion. Journal of Parasitic Diseases, 40 (4): 1116-1129.

Sharma M, Batta MK, Katoch RC, Andersen AA (2008). A field investigation of bacterial etiology of abortions among migratory sheep and goats in North-West hill states of India. Veterinarski Arhiv, 78 (1): 65-71.

Smith MC and Sherman DM (2009). Respiratory System. In: Goat Medicine. Wiley-Blackwell Publication, Iowa, 2nd edition, pp. 354-355.

Szeredi L, Jánosi S, Tenk M, Tekes L, Bozsó M, Deim Z, Molnár T (2006). Epidemiological and pathological study on the causes of abortion in sheep and goats in Hungary (1998-2005). Acta Veterinaria Hungarica, 54 (4): 503-15.

The Merck Veterinary Manual (2010). Kahn CM and Line S (Eds.). Merck & Co. Inc. (USA), Tenth Edition.

Vandyousefi D and Zoghi E (1988): Mycotic abortions in Iran. Archives de Institut-Razi, 38: 65-71.

Verma S, Katoch RC, Jand SK, Nigam P (1999). Fungi associated with abortions and infertility in does and ewes. Veterinarski Arhiv, 69(1): 1-5.

Veterinary Medicine (2000). Radostits OM, Gay CC, Blood DC and Hinchcliff KW (Eds.). ELBS Publication, London (UK), Ninth Edition.

23

Setting Up of Buck Semen Cryopreservation Laboratory

Ravi Ranjan, Manish Kumar, Praveen Kumar and Kaustubh

Division of AP&R, ICAR-Central Institute for Research on Goats, Makhdoom Mathura- 281 122, Uttar Pradesh

The major requirement that distinguishes frozen semen/IVF laboratory from other laboratories is the need to maintain aseptic conditions. The wash up and sterilization of media and other equipments should be located at one end of the room and clean area for sterilize handling at the other end, and preparation, storage and incubation in between. The storage and incubation area should be near to the sterile working area.

In recent years, the introduction of laminar flow cabinets has been a great boon in providing a sterile working area and allows the use of unspecialized laboratory accommodation for culture work. For sterile work, area should be in a quiet part of the laboratory preferably in a cubicle where a laminar flow cabinet is suitably fitted. The area should be free from dust or draughts. Nothing should be stored on the laminar flow cabinet or bench used for sterile handling except most necessary equipments like holding pipettes etc. The laminar flow cabinets provide sterile air blown over the work surface. For laboratory, a horizontal laminar flow is more preferable as opposed to a vertical one because of ease of handling the ovaries etc. If an air curtain is provided at the door of the cabinet, introduction of dust etc. can be avoided. In India laminar flow are manufactured by companies like Clenzoids, Yorco etc, among others. The laminar flow size should be a minimum of 300 X 300 or 450 X 450 mm with a 12-18 in, square filter size).

The room should be provided some amount of temperature control and dual thermostats in parallel are standard for most laboratories in the west. The door for such laboratories should be well insulated and preferably self-closing.

It may be convenient to position a bench to carry microscope etc, close to the sterile handling area, either dividing the area or separating it from other end

of the lab. The service bench should have provisions for storage of sterile glassware, plastics, pipettes, screw caps, syringes etc., in drawer units below and shelves above. The bench may also house other accessory equipments such as a small bench top centrifuge. The bench should provide a close supply of the immediate requirements.

Media preparation: The area marked for media preparation should have a coarse and fine balance, pH meter and an osmometer. Bench space will be required for dissolving and stirring solutions, and for bottling and packaging. Heat stable solutions and equipment can be autoclaved for sterilization.

Wash-up and sterilization facilities should be in a separate room outside the laboratory as the humidity and heat that they produce are difficult to dissipate. Autoclaves, ovens and distillation apparatus should be located in a separate room with an efficient exhaust fan. The wash up area should have plenty of space for soaking glassware and deep sinks for manual washing of glassware. There should be plenty of bench space for handling baskets of glassware, sorting pipettes, packaging and sealing sterile packs and a pipette washer and drier.

Storage must be provided for sterile liquids at room temperature, media at 4^0C and at -20^0C or -70^0C. Refrigerators and freezers should be located towards the nonsterile end of the laboratory. As a rough guide, you will need 200 litre for 4^0C storage and 100 L for -20^0C storage per person.

The laboratory floor should be covered with vinyl or other dust proof finish. Allow a slight fall in the level towards a floor drain located in the center of the room or on one side. This allows liberal use of water if the floor has to be washed, but more important, it protects equipment from damaging floods if stills, autoclaves or sinks overflow.

The wash up and sterilization areas can be separated, so much the better. If you have a separate wash-up and sterilization facility, it will be convenient to have this on the same floor and adjacent. Make sure that your laboratory doors are wide enough to allow entry to all the equipment you want, particularly laminar flow units, cold handling cabinets and ultra-low temperature freezers. Also allow space for maintenance.

Equipments needed for such a laboratory can be grouped in the category of essential, beneficial and useful.

Essential

Cold Handling Cabinet

Straw printing machine

Automatic Bio-Freezer

Incubator

Autoclave

Oven

Refrigerator

Freezer

Inverted microscope

Soaking bath or sink

Deep washing sink

Pippette washer

Water purifier or Water Distillation Apparatus

Bench centrifuge

Liquid nitrogen freezer

Liquid nitrogen storage cylinders

Operational Equipment

Laminar Flow Hood (Horizontal)

Cell counter

Vacuum pump

Coarse and fine balance

pH meter

Osmometer

Phase contrast microscope

Portable temperature recorder

Magnetic stirrer

Pipette dryer

Automatic pipettes or dispensers

Sterilizing oven and drying oven (separate)

Useful

-70°C freezer

Closed circuit TV

Time-lapse cinemicrographic equipment

Interference contrast microscope

Polythene bag sealer

Controlled-rate cooler

Computer

Water Purification: Water is purified for two main purposes. (1) Rinsing glassware and (2) making up media and reagent. For the first, a simple deionizer or reverse osmosis unit is adequate. For the second, higher purity water is required. The traditional method was to use double glass distilled water (glass or silica or quartz sheathed elements) but many laboratories now replace the first distillation stage with deionization. The deionizer should have a conductivity meter monitoring the effluent to signify when the cartridge must be changed and quality of water output. Deionization alone is insufficient, as many organic contaminants are not retained by the ion-exchange resins. Distillation is usually recommended as a necessary second step.

Now a days, high grade water filtration systems have become available especially Millipore etc. These filtration systems use multiple filtration techniques including high-grade deionization, charcoal filtration, reverse osmosis, ion exchange resin filtration and finally through solid state Millipore filters.

Personal Hygiene while washing etc. has been much debated but use of aprons, surgical gloves, caps, gowns and face masks are often recommended. Some of them may be absolutely necessary but others do sometime help. If you have long hair, tie it back (especially for ladies). Do not talk while working aseptically. If you have a cold do not do any tissue culture during the infection.

Standard glass or disposable plastic pipettes are easiest form of manipulating liquids. Syringes are often used but not recommended as they produce high shearing forces when dispensing cells and increase the risk of self-inoculation.

Deep screw caps should be used in preference to stoppers and when washing caps, it must be ensured that all detergent is rinsed from behind rubber liners.

The screw cap should be covered with aluminum foil to protect the neck of the bottle from sedimentary dust.

In a horizontal type of laminar flow, the air flow blows from the side facing you, parallel to the work surface and is not recirculated. In a vertical cabinet, the air blows down from the top of the cabinet on to the work surface and is either recirculated or vented.

If known human pathogens are handled, a class III pathogen cabinet with a pathogen trap on the vent is obligatory. Ultraviolet lights are used to sterilize the air and exposed work surfaces in laminar flow cabinets between use.

Biosafety and biohazards

No one should ignore potential biohazards. The most common form of injury in lab results from accidental handling of broken glass. Take care when fitting a bulb or pipetting device onto a pipette. A fire extinguisher should be wall mounted on some convenient place in the laboratory. UV light sterilization should be done with adequate protection to the skin and eyes.

24

Biosecurity Measures to be Followed in Semen Cryopreservation Laboratory Complex

S.D. Kharche, Chetna Gangwar, Ravi Ranjan, S.P. Singh and Y.K. Soni

Division of AP&R, ICAR-Central Institute for Research on Goats, Makhdoom Mathura- 281 122, Uttar Pradesh

Estimation of Bacterial Load in Buck Semen

The successful AI program depends on the health of the semen donors followed by hygiene in semen collection, processing, storage and AI methods as well as reproductive health of the females. However, the microbial contamination may not be able to avoid completely but it can be reduced to the minimum threshold level by adopting hygienic procedures.

The hygienic condition of the neat / frozen semen samples can be assessed periodically by enumerating the bacterial load apart from the periodical screening of bucks for the presence of various causative agents in animals and its transfer to the females via semen samples.

Though both viable and total (viable and nonviable) bacterial counts can be done, the viable techniques are more commonly used in diagnostic and food hygiene procedures. The viable bacteria are capable of multiplication with the production of visible colonies on or in agar media. In viable techniques, the assumption is made that one well-spaced bacterial cell gives rise to one colony. The bacterial colonies, rather than bacterial cells, are counted in these techniques. Among the viable counting techniques like Spread plate, Pour plate, Miles, Misra, Filtration are available and each has its own inherent errors, the pour plate counting method is explained as follows:

Procedure

- Ten serial dilutions of the semen samples should be made after thorough mixing of the samples using separate sterile pipettes in each transfer step. The sterile phosphate buffer saline can be used as diluent.

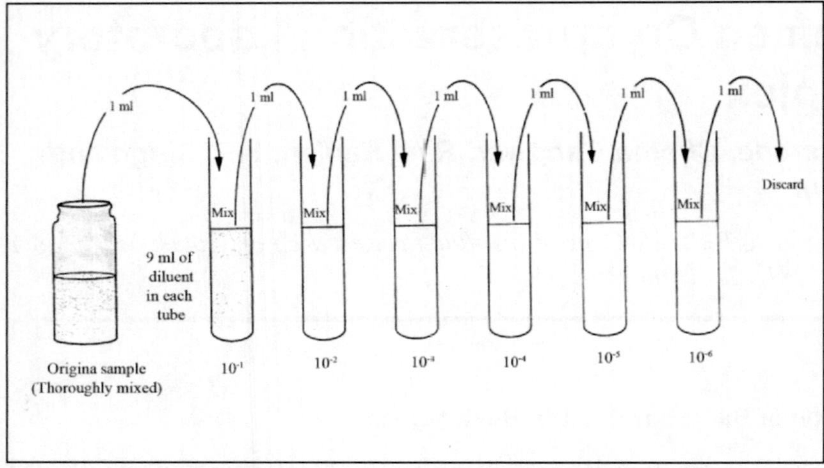

Serial Dilutions of the Semen Samples

- All the steps should be carried out aseptically and the glasswares, pipettes, agar, diluents etc. should be prepared/used after sterilization.
- The plate count agar/nutrient agar/MacConkey agar can be used for microbial growth. The agar should be prepared as per the direction of the manufacturer in the conical flask and should be autoclaved at 1200C/15 min/15lbs pressure. Then cool the agar to 45-500C by keeping the flask in water bath.
- Two to four petri plates should be inoculated for each dilution.
- Take the diluted semen samples (inoculum) at any arbitrary volume in the sterile petri plates in laminar flow and pour the agar from water bath and mix well by gently rotating the petri plates in circular motion.
- Allow the agar to set/solidify in petri plates and incubate at 25-370C for 24-48 hours.

Consider the petri plates having 30-300 colonies only for calculation of bacterial count for greatest accuracy. The colonies will be distributed throughout the agar as well as on the surface. The subsurface colonies will assume a biconvex shape.

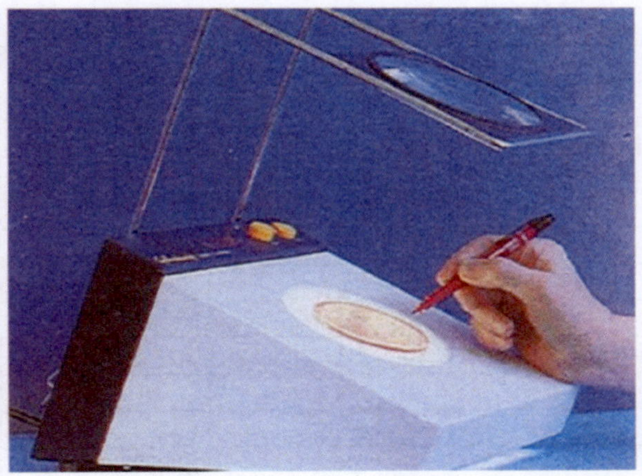

Colony Count by Electronic Counter

- The colony count should be an average of two/four plates inoculated with the selected dilution using electronic colony counter.

Calculation

Total bacterial load = Average number of colonies X reciprocal of dilution used X Quantity of inoculum used

For example,

If there is a mean count of 250 colonies at 10^{-4} dilution and the inoculum was 1.1 ml per plate, then

Number of bacteria /0.1 ml of original sample = 250 X 10^4 Number of bacteria / ml of original sample = 250 X 10^4 X 10

= 250 X 10^5

= 2.5 X 10^7 cfu/ml

Disease Transmission Status of Infective Agents in Sheep and Goat semen

Though the presence and transmission of various pathogenic organisms have been studied and demonstrated in semen of livestock in developed countries for International Trade, the same is yet to be demonstrated in India. Hence the reference of disease transmission through semen from New Zealand is given below for reference purposes.

Sr.No.	Disease or pathogenic agent	Presence	Transmission
1.	F. M. D virus	P ()	T()
2.	Rinderpest	P	T()
3.	Blue Tongue	P	T
4.	Rift valley fever	P ()	T()
5.	P. P. R	P	T()
6.	Goat pox	P	T
7.	Nairobi Sheep disease	P	LNN
8.	Wessels born disease	P	Not Transmitted
9.	Ovine pulmonary adenomatosis	P ()	T()
10.	louping-ill virus.	LNN	LNN
11.	Lentivirus/ Maedi-visna virus,	LNN	LNN
12.	Orbivirus	LNN	LNN
13.	Vesiculovirus	LNN	LNN
13.	Vesiculovirus	LNN	LNN
14.	Brucellosis (B. melitensis)	P	T()
15.	Anthrax (*Bacillus anthracis)*	N	N
16.	Mycobacterium caprae	LNN	LNN
17.	Mycobacterium paratuberculosis	P ()	T()
18.	Heart water (R. ruminantium)	Not present	-
19.	Leptospirosis (Leptospira spp.)	P	LN
20.	*Coxiella burnetti*	P	NN.
21.	Mycoplasma agalactia	P	NN.
22.	Salmonellosis (S. abortus bovis)	P	NN.
23.	Enzootic abortion of ewes (*Chlamydia psittaci*)	P	T
24.	Salmonella spp.	P ()	T()
25.	Leptospira spp.	P ()	LNN
26.	Babesia spp.	N	N
27.	Theileria spp.	N	N
28.	Trypanosome spp.	N	N
29.	Anaplasma spp.	N	N

Source: Import risk analysis: Sheep and Goat Genetic Material, Biosecurity New Zealand Ministry of Agriculture and Forestry, Wellington, New Zealand, 2005.

P: Presence demonstrated; **T:** Transmission demonstrated; **():** Non demonstrated but highly probable; **LN-** Low but non-negligible; **N-** negligible, **NN.** - non- negligible.

Safety, Precautions and Sterilization

Hygiene of the semen laboratory and sterilization of instruments, glass wares and consumables will eliminate the most of the problems that consumes valuable time and resources in this technology. Therefore, maintaining hygienic condition and proper sterilization throughout the experiment is the key for successful AI.

1. **Personnel Hygiene:** While working in the laboratory, one should wear an apron. The hands should be sterilized properly by washing with spirit.

2. **Washing and Sterilization of Equipments:** All kinds of instruments and appliances, which are required during the preparation of buffer solutions and semen extenders, and also those which are required to handle semen during dilution, storage and insemination, must be sterilized before use. It should be made a regular practice to observe aseptic precautions during any process of artificial insemination. The articles must be rinsed and washed with hot soap solution followed by distilled water. Use of corrosive, detergents should be avoided, as it may reduce the life of rubber-wares. Use of distilled water does not leave salt deposits on articles after drying. The articles should be prepared for autoclaving by closing their openings with paper. Other articles which do not have any opening, should be wrapped in paper.

3. **Artificial Vagina:** The artificial vagina should be thoroughly cleaned in hot detergent solution with a brush in order to remove all traces of grease. All rubber and polyethylene articles including artificial vagina should be autoclaved at 10Ib (4 kg) pressure (115.6^{0}C) for 20 minutes. Higher pressure may spoil the shape of these items. Other items must be autoclaved at 13 Ib (7kg) pressure (121.3^{0}C) for 15 minutes. Immediately after autoclaving, all the articles should be dried in hot air oven at 40 to 60^{0}C. Use of hot air blower at 60^{0}C may be practical in the case of rubber and paper items. Sterilized articles must be stored in air tight cabinets. Hot air oven itself may serve as a storage cabinet for all the items, but rubber items, clothes and artificial vagina should be stored in other cabinets. Paper wrappings of the articles should be removed only at the time of use, otherwise they may again be contaminated.

4. **Glassware and Metallic Ware:** Dry heat sterilization may be practiced for glass and metallic-wares. These articles should be maintained in hot air oven at 180 to 200^{0}C for one hour. If an autoclave is not available, sterilization of article should be carried out by boiling them in distilled water for 10 minutes. Use of fish kettle sterilizer is helpful for the sterilization of small items. sometimes glass-wares do not look clean and become foggy. Use of potassium dichromate solution (1%) with concentrated hydrochloric acid may be helpful to remove cloudiness from glasswares when they are treated with it.

5. **Plastic Ware:** Plastic and rubber ware can also be sterilized by gas sterilization (Ethylene oxide) so as to avoid contamination during semen processing. However as for as possible, all the sterile disposable articles should be used for semen processing.

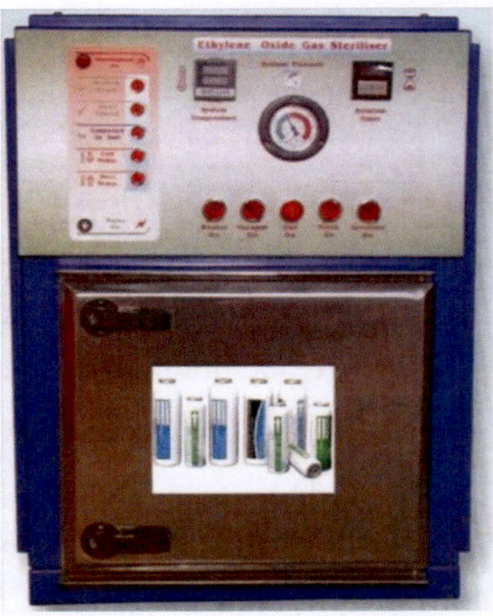

Ethylene Oxide Gas Sterilizer

6. **Tris Buffer:** The buffer used in semen laboratory is prepared hygienically. The pH (6.8) and osmolality (280-290 mOs) are adjusted before filtration. Buffer solutions and Vaseline should also be autoclaved at 15 Ib (7 kg) pressure for 15 minutes. When buffer solutions have cooled down to room temperature, they should be stored in the refrigerator for future use. The media can also be sterilized by filtration through 0.22µm filters and stored in a tightly packed sterile disposable culture vials/bottles. The media are equilibrated at least for half an hour before use in a water bath at 37°C.

7. **Laminar Flow:** The working table of laminar flow is cleaned with spirit. The laminar flow and UV tube light are put on at least half an hour before start of the work in the laminar flow.

8. **Incubator:** The incubator is sterilized with isopropyl alcohol. The stainless-steel trays are removed from the incubator. After drying all the tray, inner surfaces and corners of the incubator are cleaned and sterilized with a gauge of isopropyl alcohol. The trays are allowed to dry and then fitted in to incubator.

9. **Fumigation:** Fumigation is carried out to sterilize the semen processing laboratory and semen collection shed. A 35 mm glass petridish containing 5 gm of potassium permanganate and 10 ml of formaldehyde is put in a 90 mm glass petridish in two to four corners of the semen processing laboratory for overnight. The room is closed tightly. The formaldehyde gas released sterilize the whole semen processing laboratory. The laboratory is opened in the next morning allowing gas to pass out. The semen processing should be done at least 2-4 days after fumigation.